I0052233

The Trust Factor™

The Trust Factor™

Empowering Your Team, Your Patients,
and Your Dental Practice

Jonathan M. Abenaim D.M.D.

Copyright © 2017 by Jonathan M. Abenaim D.M.D.

All rights reserved. No part of this book may be reproduced or transmitted in any form or by any means, electronic or mechanical, including photocopying, recording, or by any information storage and retrieval system, except in the case of brief quotations embodied in critical articles and reviews, without prior written permission of the publisher.

Although the author and publisher have made every effort to ensure that the information in this book was correct at press time, the author and publisher do not assume and hereby disclaim any liability to any party for any loss, damage, or disruption caused by errors or omissions, whether such errors or omissions result from negligence, accident, or any other cause. The advice and contents in this book are the author's opinion. The author is not making any claims or promises.

Printed in the United States of America

ISBN-13 Paperback: 978-0692836309

Library of Congress Control Number: 2017900215

Cover Design: Michelle Manley
Interior Design: Ghislain Viau

Dedicated to the many people that have allowed me to do what I do every day. In no particular order, I want to thank my parents for their dedication and their tireless efforts to make sure I always had what I needed; my team who every day makes me be the best that I can be and who has taught me so much as to what it means to be a caring doctor, person and human being. Last but not least, this book is dedicated to my wife and children who never question my determined efforts and encourage me to do more and to always go beyond the status quo.

Contents

Contributions

Stephanie Curcio R.M.A. C.E.T. C.P.T.

Stephanie is the Treatment Coordinator at the Jonathan Dental Spa. She has focused her education and experience to serving in healthcare in 2009. After meeting Dr. Jonathan in 2014, her passion blossomed into creating the ultimate patient experience in dentistry. If you ask her, joining JDS was not a choice, but fate. She hails from Lancaster, PA. She is proud to be the mother of her beautiful daughter Charlotte and a blessed wife to her best friend John.

Kailey Allen R.D.H.

Kailey is the dental hygienist at Jonathan Dental Spa. She is the lead educator in the practice and prides herself on delivering the best care to her patients while educating them to understand the statuses of their oral health. She is married to her husband Mike.

Sonja Milevski R.D.A.

Sonja is the lead dental assistant at the Jonathan Dental Spa. She is the most trusted person that patients go to for confirmation and clarification on their dental treatments. She has been a dental assistant since 2001, and prides herself on enabling her patients to be comfortable, and most importantly, to receive the best treatment. She is a mom to three spectacular children: Ava, Aleksa, and Maksim. She is married to her doting husband Tommy.

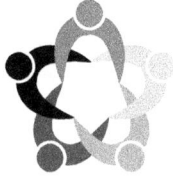

CHAPTER 1

Hey Team: *We Are All In This Together!*

Who wants to visit the dentist?

From the dentist's perspective, most patients associate a trip to the dental office with pain, money, and fear (not exactly anyone's vision of a pleasant outing). As a result, dentists believe, patients avoid their office at all costs.

So what do you do if you are the dentist? You spin the image.

If you can get people to see past the misconception of pain, money, and fear, then you can convince your patients to come in for the treatment they need. In the end, you have patients, and in return, your patients have healthy smiles.

Everyone wins, right?

Well, not quite.

The problem with this assumption—that the obstacle between your patients and your practice has everything to do with pain, money, and fear—is that it misses the point.

The reason your potential patient doesn't reach for the phone to schedule an appointment isn't because of pain, money, or fear. These could all be factors, but the overwhelming obstacle boils down to something entirely different.

The real issue is trust.

How does your office inspire trust? That is the make-or-break question.

If your patient trusts your dental hygienist, assistant, and your subsequent team members—and your dental hygienist, assistant, and team members trust you—then you create a circle of trust and communication that empowers everyone to feel fulfilled and satisfied.

If your patients trust your office, then they believe that the service you provide is in their best interest and they will keep coming back to you for treatment.

If the team trusts the dentist, then the office functions as a cohesive whole. Nothing can prevent you from achieving a tremendous amount of success, and a solid patient foundation.

Why is this idea of "trust" so important? Quite simply, the dental business is not like it used to be.

Once upon a time, a dental practice was a staple of the community. Oral health is fundamental to overall health; therefore, the dental practice could only succeed. You could practically hang a shingle outside and be instantly successful, with a busy practice.

Today, it's a different story. The dental practice can no longer ride the tide of economic downturns. In the past decade, individual practices have gone the same way as mom-and-pop traditional businesses: there is no guarantee that customers will keep coming back.

Traditional business models and methodologies cannot compete with the modern market. Those practices that cannot adapt will sink to the bottom, while the offices that think to the future will survive—and thrive. Most importantly, the so-called "competition" will be left in the dust.

Service to patients is the same, but operations within a firm—the core values and metrics—are key to surviving in today's world. The Trusted Dental™ office must have its vision set before they even begin. As Stephen Covey would say, "Begin with the end in mind."

Gone is the top-down dictatorship. Today, the dental office is a true democracy. Like any democracy, the dental practice must be governed by a kind and benevolent leader who inspires—that's right—*trust*.

The modern dental practice thrives on trust.

Stop believing the dentist is a stand-alone company. Instead, embrace, build, and maintain a true team. Grow your business by growing trust.

Consider a rowing team. Each person at his or her oar must work together to synchronize every stroke for maximum speed and efficiency. The better the team can row together, the more precisely they coordinate their strokes and the closer they will come to winning the race.

A rowing team cannot lead itself. On the contrary, the team relies upon a coxswain to count the strokes and ensure everyone is rowing in time. The coxswain wouldn't get anywhere without his or her skilled rowers, nor would the rowers know where to go—or have the fortitude to keep rowing, come what may—without the coxswain at the helm.

Your dental practice is the boat. If everyone is rowing the same way, on the same boat, then the company can crush the competition in any market, in any business, at any time.

No one can avoid the occasional roadblock, but if everyone is on the same page, problems can be solved faster, and much more easily.

To Be a True Leader, Take off the Mask

The definition of a leader is not someone who tells you what to do. A leader is someone who makes you feel better about yourself whenever you're around him or her. A leader is someone who inspires trust.

So many practices fail because the doctor cannot see beyond the treatment room. They forget that they are leaders and instead see themselves more like the Lone Ranger, charging through rocky terrain to rescue the patient in distress.

The Lone Ranger would have made a lousy dentist.

The Lone Ranger works alone (aside from his sidekick and trusty steed), and so he couldn't empower the very key to a successful dental practice: his people.

The implicit message here is that a leader works *with people*. As a dentist, you are the leader of your practice. In order to lead, you must take off the mask and embrace your people.

This book isn't just for the dentist. This book is for every member of the team.

Throughout this book, you will hear firsthand accounts from a dentist, dental assistant, dental hygienist, and treatment care coordinators; every member of the office who is involved in treating patients and making sure the process is smooth, efficient, and enjoyable. This book has contributions from the whole Trusted Dental™ team, because we believe that the cohesive team is the key to the dream practice. Once that is in place, the rest is simple.

The doctor will better understand how to empower his or her team because he or she will better understand the role that each member in the office plays, along with his or her unique needs and desires.

All team members will learn how to empower themselves, work well with their teammates, and feel incredibly satisfied and fulfilled with the work that they do.

You will also learn about the view from the dental chair. Your patients have an oar on your boat, so don't make any assumptions about what your patients want or need. Develop those factors with them. Gather the clues they drop in relation to money, treatment, and fear (more on that later in the book).

The practice's success depends on the team's ability to inspire trust in the patient.

The success of your team building trust and calming the patient is your ability to lead and empower your people.

We have a process that inspires trust. In this book, we will show you how to incorporate it into your own practice.

We will show you how—if you can teach your team members to do *their* best, and convince your patient that *you* will do *your* best while treating her like family—you will have knocked down the biggest obstacle to treating your patient.

Once you have the clues and keys to the problem, you can solve any problem that arises with your patients or your team.

Together, you will all learn to row—and grow—as one cohesive team.

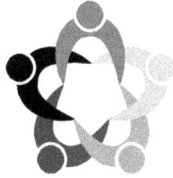

CHAPTER 2

Dear Dental Assistant: Become the It

With Contributions from
Sonja Milevski, RDA, CTF-DA

A quick Google search will tell you that a dental assistant is responsible for helping the dental operator provide more efficient dental treatment. It will also tell you that a surgeon is a specialist in any treatment that involves the cutting of a body.

What do these two descriptions have in common? They both fall drastically short of conveying what the people in these positions *actually do.*

Many dentists are guilty of the same error. They see their assistants as people who are there to help with procedures and preparations, but they fail to see beyond this very limiting description. Don't get us wrong; dentists all understand the value of the dental assistant. Whether they really understand the *value* of the CTF-DA ("Certified Trust Factor Dental Assistant™") is yet to be determined.

This oversight may not seem like a big deal, but it could actually be costing your practice in time, money, and patients.

How does a three-day work week sound to you? What about increased autonomy, job satisfaction, and success?

To many people, this sounds like a dream-job scenario, but I'm here to tell you, it exists. In a Trust Factor™ office, trust can turn the practice into a dream job for everyone. It begins with understanding what a dental assistant can do for you.

Most offices don't recognize the full potential of their dental assistants. As a result, they underutilize their skills and hinder what could be a building block of the practice.

To the dental assistant reading this: I want you to learn to feel empowered, nurtured, and to ask for more—because you deserve more. You should feel awesome about what you provide and accomplish every day.

To the dentist: This chapter will help you understand how to help your assistant attain this level of confidence and autonomy.

The Gatekeeper

As you train to become a dental assistant, you learn all about what to expect on the job, from suctioning to setting up and caring for the patient.

Now I want you to imagine being a contestant on *The Price Is Right*. Just as the host reveals the grand prize, Bob Barker cuts in: "But wait; there's more!"

That's right, there is so much more to being a dental assistant. You just might not know it unless you work in a Trust Factor™ office and become a CTF-DA.

In a Trust Factor™ office, you're not just a dental assistant; you're the gatekeeper. From the patient's standpoint, you are the most trusted person in the office. Hence, the Dental Assistant chapter is first in the layout of this book.

Many patients, whether we realize it or not, would love to have comprehensive care. They haven't been to the dentist in years, most likely for the very reason that they weren't sure they could trust someone with the dental work they needed. Now that they are in the office, they are scared. Building trust is everything.

In the patient's eyes, the dentist is the one who performs the treatment with his frightening instruments. To him or her, the dentist is authoritative and down-to-business, which is OK. After all, you want the person holding the drill to appear as if he knows what he's doing. However, the consequence of this "authoritative" perception is that patients can be scared to tell the doctor just how they feel.

Although the dentist performs the operations, he is often the person in the office with whom the patient has the least communication. The patient doesn't always feel as comfortable sharing his or her insecurities or concerns with the doctor.

With the dental assistant, the patient is less embarrassed and more likely to share. By the time you get to the treatment process, you've established a rapport with the patient. As you go through transformations and procedures, you take time to ask every so often how the patient is doing, knowing that he or she is more likely to communicate with you.

At the end of it all, when you hand over the mirror and the patient sees his or her new smile, it's the most rewarding feeling of all—something money couldn't buy. It wouldn't happen, however, if you didn't inspire the trust of the patient, and if the dentist didn't establish trust with you. As the CTF-DA, you are as much a part of that life-changing event as the doctor. Don't sell yourself short. You are important and vital to the machine.

A lot of dentists and dental assistants don't realize that the assistant is the most trusted person in the office. We have interviewed and asked hundreds of DAs about who they thought was most trusted, and we have the data to prove it. Very few were aware of how vital they were within the office. Most assistants felt overworked, underpaid, and underappreciated. By recognizing this relationship, the doctor can help to give the patient a voice through the assistant, and ultimately, allow the whole team to win.

So how do you, the dental assistant (or the gatekeeper), inspire trust?

The Trust Handoff™

Trust begins with the dentist internally. He has to take the first step with being able to create trust in his office by trusting his team. In a Trust Factor™ office, the doctor trusts the assistant to take on responsibility and inspires her to be better each day. That effect really comes across to the patients and factors into how the assistant interacts with the patients.

In the same way that the doctor treats the assistant as an equal, the assistant treats the patients as equals.

Each time a new patient comes in, prior to the doctor seeing her, the assistant and treatment coordinator conduct a pre-interview with her. At this stage, the concern is not so much her dental history; rather, the goal is to get to know more about her and what led her to the office. What made her do what she's doing at this point in her life? Does she have any important events coming up? The Trust Factor™ practice has an agreement with its team members: do not speak about treatment with any patient until you know five things about her.

To be clear: the assistant doesn't talk *to* the patient; the assistant talks *with* the patient. You sit right next to her, on the same level, eye to eye, knee to knee, and stay with her the whole time. Do not stand on top of her. Do not stand behind her. Speak to her as if she were the last person you would speak to in your life. Give her the utmost respect.

The CTF-DA never leaves the patient alone in the dental chair. You would never want to be left alone in a room prior to making a decision that would involve time, money, and something you may not think you need. You can now begin to start your record-taking. You reassure the patient as you take intraoral pictures. Guide her through the process. Speak to her to make her feel comfortable. After all that, you can review the data and show her what could be going on. You're not diagnosing; essentially, you're "making her aware" and initiating the education process before the doctor comes in.

So what is this "Trust Handoff™" we are talking about? The treatment care coordinator does the first brief interview, and then she hands off trust to the assistant. The assistant has the first opportunity to really get to know the patient as a person and gain her trust. Once you get that trust from her, you hand off to the doctor.

The assistant is with the patient when the doctor goes over the treatment. When the doctor steps out, the assistant asks the patient, "Did he answer everything correctly? Do you have any concerns? Is this what you want?" The doctor puts trust in the assistant to allow the patient to trust the team. What this also accomplishes is leveraging the position of the dental assistant in the trust hierarchy by empowering her to be with the patient prior to any monetary discussion.

Patients don't come into a Trust Factor™ office solely to be sold on the best technology. They couldn't care less what model of equipment is in the room. What they really want to know is, *Can I trust this person to perform the treatment that I need?*

This is vastly different from most other dental offices, where assistants remain silent most of the time. In a Trust Factor™ office, the doctor gives his team the opportunity to be involved with, and have a say in, interacting with the patient for her clinical needs. He allows the assistant to make that first connection, which a lot of offices don't do. As a result, those "other offices" are underutilizing their best line of trust to the patient: the CTF-DA.

The Trust Handoff™ also allows the team to really treat each patient. They don't run through the appointment list as quickly as possible. Rather, they take the time to educate the patient about her dental health and how it connects to the rest of her life. A typical dental office can spend 90 percent of the time worrying about 10 percent of the patients. The Trust Factor™ office aims to change that reality.

In a Trust Factor™ office, the doctor realizes that if the patient doesn't trust the team, then she's not going to come back. No matter what, if the patient needs treatment, she will try to find the money. But if she doesn't trust the team, she's not having them do the work.

Trust the Team

The message in other offices is, "The dentist cannot trust his team members." So why should the patients trust the team?

It comes down to validation. When a dentist fails to recognize the full potential of his dental assistant, then he is holding her back. Good things come when someone is validated. Validation makes one feel empowered to do more than he or she might normally do.

The doctor validates the team by giving them the freedom to help educate the patients. Positive affirmations provide a tremendous confidence booster and fosters goodwill within the office.

In Gary Chapman's book, *The 5 Love Languages*®, the author mentions that in the workplace, "we don't call them the 5 *love* languages; rather, we call them the *appreciation* languages. Consider them like family members—similar, but not exactly . . . the nature of work-based relationships." When the Trust Factor™ office team knows each other's appreciation languages, getting people to their best potential is all downhill.

In a Trust Factor™ office, the doctor knows that if you're not happy with what you do, it's going to be apparent in your work. That discontentment is going to show, and even the patient is going to realize, *This is not the place for me.*

On the other hand, if you truly love what you do, then that love is conveyed to the patient. Patients can read your body language in the office. You may think you are faking it and doing fine. Consider that every one of your patients is a body-language expert. Do you want to work in an environment where it doesn't matter what people think because you love, and are the best at, what you do?

When the patient sees how much you love what you do, then the message she receives is, *These people really care about me.*

More than "Just" a Job

A Trust Factor™ office inspires the team to learn and grow beyond the job description because of the positive dynamic the doctor establishes in the office. When someone trusts you with their livelihood and their practice, then you feel good about what you do.

This growth extends to your personal life, as well. Sometimes people leave their job at the end of the day and put it out of sight, out of mind. The Trust Factor™ team members take what they learn from the job and bring it into their personal lives to better every aspect of life outside work. That inspiration to become a better person carries over from your professional life with your Trust Factor™-empowered doctor. Being a dental assistant is not "just" a job; it's a journey.

Incentivizing the Team

Not only does the dentist empower his team, but the team empowers the dentist as well. The Trust Factor™ doctor knows that although his name is on the door, you are all equal partners in the success of the practice. He emphasizes this factor by rewarding his team when they help grow the business. When the dentist grows emotionally, professionally, and financially, everyone grows.

The doctor can incentivize his team members in multiple ways to become better at what they do. A bonus system does not exist in a Trust Factor™ office; rather, a partnership system is in place. Your Trust Factor™ team members are your partners in everything you do. Treat them as such— financially, emotionally, and respectfully.

It's a rare occurrence to hear about offices that recognize their employees with a reward for going above and beyond. Most dentists are afraid that incentivizing employees translates to losing money. In the Trust Factor™ office, this has the opposite effect. By incentivizing, the team brings in more business and retains more business.

Work Smart

Most offices are open five or six days a week, sometimes including Saturdays, but not the Trust Factor™ practice. In just three days, the Trust Factor™ practice is able to do what other full-time offices do. This true balance allows the doctor and the team to have lives outside of the office. Whether it is raising a family, giving back to the community, accepting teaching assignments, or just having FUN, it can all be accomplished in a three-day workweek.

When speaking of success, a common maxim is "Work smarter, not harder." Well, the Trust Factor™ practice *does* work hard, but in a different way.

Compared to that of other dental assistants, the scope of the work is probably more intense. However, the Trust Factor™ assistant takes on more responsibility because she loves her job, and because she loves it, she accomplishes so much more.

The Trust Factor™ team achieves success with a three-day workweek because the doctor uses all of his team members to their full potential. He trusts the team and treats them as equals, and everyone works together to accomplish amazing things.

When each person does what she needs to do, and is empowered to go above and beyond what she's actually expected to do, then all of the team members perform to their fullest potential. The dental assistant isn't just there to assist; she's there to help educate the patient. And she does it just three days a week!

Other dentists are afraid. Out of fear, they don't allow their team members to work at their full potential—fear that delegating responsibility is akin to giving up control, and if someone else has control, then the whole ship could sink. Really, the dentist is placing too much responsibility on his own shoulders.

When the dentist sits down with his patients to review treatment—work that could be done by the assistant—he is taking time away from other duties in which he might be better utilized. By allowing the assistant to help manage his time and educate the patient with her treatments, the assistant makes his job easier, as well that of the rest of the team. The doctor should have a scalpel, drill, explorer, curing light, or any other fun tool in his hand—not a keyboard or a pen. Tasks that utilize the latter can be delegated to others who are more trained than he is at accomplishing them.

Who wouldn't want to work fewer days, all the while making more money than in a traditional five-day workweek? When you really break it down, there isn't anyone who wouldn't want to use trust to maximize his or her practice's potential. Making money is not the primary goal, but rather, having fun and changing people's lives. The money will come; it always does. The fun and the impact on people does not always manifest if it is not engraved upon your vision.

A Happy Office Is a Successful Office

One of the first things that a patient says to the dental assistant is, "I hate coming here."

After working through the Trust Handoff™ and performing treatments, you will hear it time and time again: "I love you guys!"

The patient's attitude completely changes. She's no longer afraid of the dentist; on the contrary, she loves coming in because she knows she will be cared for. Not only have you gained her trust clinically, but you've gained her trust emotionally, as well.

The Trust Factor™ practice is a second home. If you're just picking up this book, realize that you're not just your job title. You are so much more.

As a dental assistant, you're not only the dentist's helper; you're also an educator, a team member, and a counselor.

You provide excellent service to your patients, and in a Trust Factor™ office, you can make a great living working just three days a week along the way. Most importantly, you leave a legacy to what you have accomplished and have a great time doing so.

That's right; you can do it too. You can have it all, as long as you have trust.

When you inspire trust in anyone—whether it be patient, assistant, dentist, or otherwise—that individual will exceed your expectations and will love coming in to do what he or she does best.

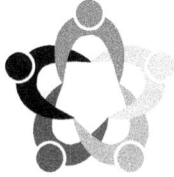

CHAPTER 3

Dear Dental Assistant: Know Your Worth (You Are My Right Hand)

With Contributions from
Sonja Milevsky, RDA, CTF-DA

"Freedom" is often one of dental assistants' last words used to describe their job. In most offices, the role is dictated by the doctor. You are there to support him, and do as he says. While that support is a very important aspect of being a dental assistant, without freedom, the doctor is only limiting himself, and the practice.

I have had the privilege of seeing both sides of the spectrum. I know what it means to have a role that is largely controlled by another person; I also know what it is like to be given the freedom to do my job and make decisions based on my experience and expertise in the Trust Factor™ office.

The difference between the two scenarios isn't just personal happiness and job satisfaction. It's also a reflection of the state of the practice.

By the end of this chapter, you will understand exactly what I mean. You will discover how empowering your team members with freedom can transform the practice and allow assistants to feel more validated and incredibly satisfied.

Life at "Other" Practices

At other practices, the assistant is a "spit sucker/vacuumer" and background support. You don't interact much with the patients because the doctor does most of the talking. In fact, the doctor does most of everything, from billing to scheduling, and, oh yeah, dentistry, too. The common side effect here is that the dentist is overworked and overstressed, and the assistant is frustrated because she could be doing so much more.

Life at the Trust Factor™ Practice

As a dental assistant at a Trust Factor™ practice, you are an educator. You educate patients about their oral health and why their mouth is so important for their overall health. You're only able to do so because the doctor grants you that freedom. He knows what an asset you are because of the amount of time you spend with the patient, building her trust.

At a Trust Factor™ office, the assistant will gain deeper insight into what makes her role effective and important. It comes together in what I call the "Rules of Engagement" for educating and gaining the trust of the patient.

The Dental Assistant's Three Rules of Engagement

1. Take the time.

When you meet with a patient, you take intraoral pictures, sit with her, and show her the pictures that depict what's going on inside her mouth. It sounds simple enough, but this kind of patient engagement is a rarity. Why? Because you're simply not given the time.

Most practices spend about thirty minutes with a new patient to educate her on her oral health. The Trust Factor™ office schedules a full hour, sometimes more. That way, you have plenty of time to connect.

Most practices might read this and think, "What?! You waste a full hour? What if she cancels?"

The proof is in the pudding, and judging by the Trust Factor™ practices' success since making the switch, an hour for each patient makes a huge difference. (I'll go into further detail about why this is the case later in this chapter.)

2. Don't talk numbers.

I mentioned before that, from the patient's standpoint, the dental assistant is the most trusted person in the office. You are with the patient the most, and so she looks to you when she has questions or concerns.

Some practices use this time to talk money—a big no-no. Discussing the financial aspects of treatment with the patient while she is comprehending what she needs for her health makes her feel uneasy and could ultimately scare her off.

You never want to risk your standing in the trust hierarchy by connecting money and education. Remember, the patient is the body-language expert. She wants to know that you are there to help her and benefit her, not the other way around. In the spirit of John F. Kennedy, a successful person asks not what can be done for him, but what he can do for others.

3. Engage.

In the Trust Factor™ office, you want to hold the patient's hand, so to speak, and make the experience as enjoyable as possible. The patient starts with the treatment coordinator, who walks the patient through the office and essentially welcomes her into our home. We remove the sense of uncertainty. Then she is introduced to the assistant.

As you take pictures, make conversation, inquire about the patient and her life, and discuss anything that may be important to her. After taking intraoral photos, point out conditions or issues that she may have. For instance, if the patient has plaque or visual issues that you and she can see, you might explain to her what is going on. Sometimes, she will be scared by what she sees. She might look away from the screen with a look of sheer terror. She may even say, "I don't even want to look at this." This is a great opportunity to reinforce that your team can help her and is there for her.

When a patient is in your care, she is in a vulnerable position. This is your opportunity to put her at ease, to tell her that although it may seem bad, it is nothing that you haven't seen before. She is with you now and you can help fix her problem. You are there for her and will be by her side throughout the whole process.

Freedom Means Having Time

In my Rules of Engagement, I listed time as an important factor; that is, in order to engage and educate the patient, and form a relationship of trust, you must give her enough time.

Most doctors see time as a cost. They think quantity will drive production, whereas *quality* is truly the key. So you you work less and are rewarded more.

The Trust Factor™ office, however, gives the dental assistant and hygienist ample time to gain the patient's trust. This time allows both team members to feel confident because they can execute their job to its fullest potential. At the same time, they are able to educate the patient about the condition of her mouth so that by the time the doctor comes in, she already understands that the dental treatment is indeed necessary.

"And what if the new patient cancels? That's two hours down the drain!" you think.

True, cancellations are an issue, especially if you don't know the patient and haven't yet formed that connection with her. So we developed a solution.

The typical office might have a new patient go through hygiene on her first visit, but sometimes patients cancel and the hygienist loses that hour.

The Trust Factor™ office filters new patients differently. Instead of having the new patient get her teeth cleaned, you conduct an initial consultation. If you determine that she needs her teeth cleaned, then you schedule an appointment for that. Once you have made that connection with the patient, you have built mutual trust that plays a huge hand in eliminating such cancellations. If a new patient doesn't show up for a consultation, then he or she will be a definite no-show for hygiene.

At the end of the initial consultation, sometimes the patient books, sometimes she doesn't. But you must always tell her that if she doesn't choose your office, you want her to be educated. It drives home the message that many practices don't necessarily care about patients' oral health, but really, just want their business. That's what makes the Trust Factor™ office different.

You may be thinking, *This sounds great, but we can't do this because [fill in the blank].* An excuse is just a well-planned lie. Everyone can do it. Maybe not exactly as prescribed, but perhaps your office can create a variation so that it works for your workflow. There will be roadblocks throughout the process until you learn to execute. This is where the Trust Factor™ training team can help you create a plan to make this possible in your office.

It may sound like a challenge, but really, transforming your practice with the Trust Factor™ in mind is your best bet for success. Trust Factor™ practices are successful because they give their all to every patient who walks through the door. Sure, they may not win them all, but a majority of them say YES, and those who do become patients for life.

Freedom Means Making Decisions

In order for the office to be successful, the assistant must be at liberty to make decisions based on her expertise and training to the doctor's standard. A lot of those decisions come down to time. How much time needs to be spent on a patient for her particular needs?

The dental assistant must be able to manage her time and schedule. The doctor may have input as to how much time something will require, but sometimes the assistant has more insight, simply because she's going through the procedures with the patients.

In other words, doctors, it's time to let go.

Once the assistant has worked alongside the doctor, she knows how the doctor works. The assistant is aware of how to best support her leader, but can only do so if the doctor lets go and trusts the assistant.

It may be scary to imagine telling your boss to "let go." If you have any hesitation about discussing these methods of empowerment with your doctor, here are some selling points to outline:

1. Trust saves time for the doctor.

Most dentists are tired of delegating. It's their practice, and they micromanage everything from assisting to the front desk and insurance. It is their livelihood, but ours, as well. This kind of responsibility takes a toll on the doctor.

The doctor has to have trust in the team members and allow them to take control. When the doctor comes in, he wants to do dentistry. That's all. The doctor doesn't want to say, "Why isn't my room ready?" or "Why didn't you collect money before the patient came in?" Trusting the team eliminates this worry and saves the doctor time.

2. Trust brings in more business for the doctor.

When the doctor trusts his teammates to perform and make decisions on behalf of the practice, it serves as an incredible incentive for the team to accomplish goals. Every person feels valued because he or she is given responsibility. That translates to greater patient satisfaction and financial success.

3. Trust spares the doctor stress.

Empowering the team is not only financially more lucrative, but it's better psychologically and emotionally as well. The doctor can come in and do what needs to be done. When he takes a much-deserved vacation, he can leave with the peace of mind that everything will be taken care of while he's away.

The Trust Factor™ doctor can truly unplug without the stress of wondering if his business will be OK. He knows it will because he trusts the team members and trusts that they care about the practice as much as he does. The whole team feels ownership because he gives them that responsibility.

The Transformative Power of Giving Trust

When you train to work at a dental practice, you may think that your education culminates when you get the job.

If you are part of a Trust Factor™ practice that empowers you with trust, then the education has only just begun. The lessons you learn, as well as the personal victories you accomplish at work, trickle into your personal life. In this day and age, when work and personal life are traditionally separated, it's wonderful to have two things that enhance all aspects of life.

By acknowledging his teammates and letting them know that they're important and he couldn't be successful without them, the doctor accomplishes a huge feat: he's letting go. Through the years, this will prove to be a transformative decision.

As a business, you want the people who work for you to feel like it's theirs too. Once they feel that way, they'll love coming to work.

It's hard to let go of control, but the reward is that at the end of the month, the Trust Factor™ office hits its goal. At the end of the month, the doctor (along with his team) can go on vacation and know their office is covered.

You will have some team members who soar and rise above and beyond; you will have others who throw in the towel, which is good because that means they're not the right team member for the office. In the Trust Factor™ office, people do not get fired; rather, they deselect themselves. It is soon obvious that being in a winning environment is not what they enjoy. The "Debbie Downers" and the "Negative Nancys'" can't handle the positive energy and hard work that is engrained in the Trust Factor™ office.

It's a process to put this in place, but even if it's a slow process, it could be a slow process *to get to where you need to be.* Sometimes the dentist has to take a step back to let his team shine through.

Each member of the Trust Factor™ team is good at what he or she does. But they are all really good at it because their dentist allows them to be good at what they do. He trusts the team members and lets them be those people. Ask your doctor for his trust in you to take steps toward attaining the validation you deserve.

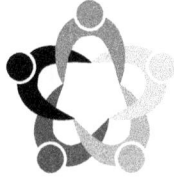

CHAPTER 4

Dear Dental Hygienists:
Work Smarter Not Harder

With Contributions from
Kailey Allen, RDH

So you decided to be a dental hygienist. Now what? You are probably all about prevention and it carries out in your job. You're dedicated to preventing disease in all aspects of life, and finding a way to be the healthiest that you can be. Congrats! You picked the perfect field.

You are passionate about preventing disease in all aspects of life, and determining a way to get your patients healthy is your goal. Now, let's teach you the Trust Factor™ way so that you can be even more successful.

Medications are being sold en masse, and while they may have lifesaving properties, they also have so many side effects. What I find interesting is that many of the conditions patients are treated for—high blood pressure, high cholesterol, diabetes, and other ailments—have manifestations in the mouth.

Being a dental hygienist means that you can help educate patients about what role their mouths play in their overall health. What most patients don't realize is that a majority of ailments are preventable if we make small lifestyle modifications. In addition to keeping a patient's mouth clean, dental hygienists have a tremendous opportunity to educate patients on matters that could improve their comprehensive health.

So how do you make that happen? How can you educate while you have patients stacked up and not enough time in the day to put in the work and give attention to each patient?

Just like that old saying goes, "Work smarter, not harder." This chapter is all about how the hygienist can empower herself by identifying key opportunities to work smart.

The Trust Factor™ practice runs off the dental hygienist's schedule. The hygienist assesses, but why do all that if the patient doesn't understand what you're doing, or why?

How many times have you spoken to a patient and she crossed her arms while she was listening? Did she even look you in the eye as you were attempting to educate her?

Were you sitting or standing in front of her, or behind her? You are on stage and your patient is your audience. Keep her engaged, and keep her asking for more.

Part of the hygienist's job is tracking data. The collection of data isn't just to fill up the chart, but instead, to educate the patient. That means you are on the frontline of informing patients on treatments that may benefit them. This aspect of the job might make you feel uncomfortable—more like a treatment salesperson than a dental hygienist. At the Trust Factor™ practice, you'll realize that you're presenting legitimate treatment that the patient needs. You can't force the patient to utilize a service, but you're doing a disservice to the patient if you don't present what is needed.

You are the only health-care practitioner in the world who spends a minimum of two full hours with a patient per year, and sometimes more. Your patient trusts you, so why would you shortchange her health? Give the patient what she deserves and what she is there for. She trusts you.

You're not selling treatment; you're *sharing* the information that you have with patients. Sharing information with people is very common. You do it every day via text messaging, Facebook, or a casual coffee date. What people choose to do with the information you share is up to them.

The Hygienist as the Caregiver

Part of the hygienist's job satisfaction is being able to help people beyond simply cleaning their teeth.

A lot of times, hygienists may feel limited by the supervision of the dentist. Maybe the dentist doesn't trust the hygienist to interact with the patient in an educational way.

Legally, hygienists have certain parameters that prevent them from diagnosing a condition. However, you collect data and information, and put the pieces of the puzzle together. You can't diagnose, but you can help to educate the patient and explain factors that may relate to whatever it is she is experiencing.

The Hygienist as the Friend

In the traditional office, the hygienist cleans teeth and calls the doctor in for an exam. If the patient has major cavities, you'll give her an appointment to come back, but beyond that, it's pretty cut and dried.

Let's face it: we are gum gardeners. At least, that's the stereotype. But really, we're so much more. Our career entails far more than that. In the Trust Factor™ office, cleaning teeth is 10 percent of what we do, while 90 percent is sharing information and educating the patient.

At the Trust Factor™ office, the hygienist does so much more. Educating your patients is very important. They need to know how often they need to come in, how we can help them, and how they can help themselves.

Like all members of the team, the hygienist works on establishing a relationship with the patients. One thing that you can do to aid in this process is greet the patient when she arrives. Always try to be very friendly and introduce yourself if she doesn't know who you are.

It is incredibly important for a dental hygienist to be friendly because the patient is in a very vulnerable situation. Most patients are terrified to even *be* at the dentist's office. You need to make them feel as comfortable as possible, and that comes across through genuine warmth and friendliness the moment you tell them you'll be taking care of their teeth.

What's the PM?

Every new patient has a personal motivator, or "PM," when he or she comes in—a reason why he or she needs treatment in the first place.

A personal motivator is more specific than whether or not one is in pain. For instance, if someone comes in for major dentistry and mentions that her grandchild asked, "How come your teeth are so yellow?" you realize that her motivator is very personal. It's cosmetic.

Usually, the PM is identified before she even gets to the hygienist. You can always keep that piece of information in the back of your mind and use her personal motivator to help connect to her. The power of the PM will come into play when a patient says no to treatment that you recommend. Reminding her of why she initially came in for treatment will place her back on the right track. At our institute, we teach the power of the PM within the patient experience.

All-Star Attitude

The Trust Factor™ doctor believes he's the best dentist, you're the best dental hygienist, he has the best dental assistant, and so on. Those are the kind of people the doctor wants to be around: people who are the best at what they do. More importantly, you can be great at what you do, but if pride is not a part of the equation, then it is all for nothing. The patient can sense that "aura" in the office and wants to be a part of it. It exudes the essence of a leader, and people crave the opportunity to be around leaders.

The Trust Factor™ office utilizes peer evaluations to stay on the same page with the rest of the team. Some questions to be asked include:

"Is this person trustworthy?"
"Is this person organized?"
"Is this person respectful of others' workspace?"

Everybody on the team rates each other and then you all sit down and go over the questions. In other offices, the dentist may just do evaluations for his "employees." In a Trust Factor™ office, employees do not exist and staff members (more like "staph infection") do not exist, but team members and partners *do*. In the Trust Factor™ office, the team reviews the dentist as well. The trusting doctor welcomes feedback—both positive and constructive.

The Trust Factor™ office does a lot of team building and self-reflection. As a result, everyone is on the same playing field and that makes it fun to go to work. Work transcends into personal life. You'll find yourself looking at other aspects of your life and wondering, "What else can I improve?"

PCS (Problem, Consequence, Solution)

Dentistry must be presented in a simple form that will allow the patient to make the correct decision about her specified treatment. A lot of patients are extremely taken aback when they are told that they need a crown, a filling, an implant, etc. Presenting the treatment to the patient in a manner in which she can understand and own her problem enables the team to gain the patient's trust, and more importantly, to help her get healthy.

When the doctor meets with you and the patient, you come up with a PCS: problem, consequence, and solution. You want to tie the PCS to the patient's personal motivator, what's driving her to take action with her dentistry. The problem could be that she has a cavity. The consequence is that the tooth will decay and eventually die. The solution is to fill the cavity.

It is of the utmost importance to follow the process the way that it is designed. We know dentists like to make it their own. This process has been tried, tested, and proven. As Marcus Lemonis from *The Profit* says, "PEOPLE, PROCESS, PRODUCT." You can't be successful without a process. As a dental office, if we have the right people (the Trust Factor™ Team), we have the right process (the Trust Factor™), and we have a great product (dental skills), then success is sure to happen.

You can use the PCS to educate the patient. The patient needs to hear the PCS five times in order to make the message sink in. The first time the patient hears her problem is from the hygienist. The second time is when the doctor comes in for the exam and the hygienist relays that information. The third time is when the doctor repeats the patient's problem to her. The fourth time is when the hygienist calls in the treatment care coordinator.

The treatment care coordinator then takes the patient from the room for treatment and brings her into the New-Life Room (we don't like the word "consultation" as it contains that negative "con"). The New-Life Room is where the coordinator repeats the problem, consequence, and solution. Repeating the PCS those five times makes a huge difference at the finish line.

In a typical dental office, the hygienist often isn't empowered to let the patient know that she may have a cavity because, again, hygienists cannot diagnose. In the Trust Factor™ office, you can point out if an area looks suspicious or concerning and have the doctor come in and confirm.

In other offices, hygienists may not feel as comfortable saying anything at all because they can't diagnose or the doctor doesn't want them to say anything. In still other offices, the hygienist just doesn't care to do that. They just clean teeth and go on—not because they don't want to say anything, but rather, because they are not empowered to do so. A hygienist is a vital part of your Trust Factor™ team. A hygienist will spend a substantial amount of time with a patient, and all of a sudden the doctor comes in for a couple minutes and says, "OK, you need two fillings and a crown. We'll see you soon."

The patient didn't hear it from the hygienist with whom she just spent a good deal of time. The doctor simply came in and rushed through it. From the patient's standpoint, the doctor isn't concerned about her health, but instead, just making money off his dentistry. The PCS process prevents this misperception.

Also, the patient could miss out on the consequences of ignoring the problem. That could amount to more pain and more money. The consequences of not treating the problem, and not educating the patient, could be serious.

Empowering the hygienist allows her to do good work and to work smarter. It also guides the patient toward the help she needs. In the end, you change people's lives, and grow into a greater version of yourself. Who could ask for more?

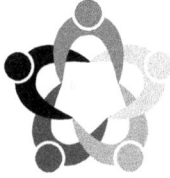

CHAPTER 5

Dear Dentist: Prioritize Time with Patients

*With Contributions from
Kailey Allen, RDH*

Whether you have a half an hour or a full hour with a patient, you still have to work smart to get everything done within the given time frame. In the previous chapter, I outlined what "working smart" looks like for the dental hygienist. In this chapter, I'll dive into how you can maximize your time with the patient. Every session is the opportunity to build trust, build a relationship, and build the good health of the patient. Let's discover how.

Connecting with the Patient

A big part of your job is taking notes. You take notes on every aspect of the patient's treatment and health, but the smart clinician will even record notes that aren't necessarily clinical. For instance, if the patient shares that her father is in the hospital, write that down. That way, the next time you see her, you can ask, "How is your father doing?"

It's a thoughtful touch, and so easy for you to do. Patients don't realize that you're just writing in a chart. They think that you genuinely remember when they come in.

Send a Note

There are so many simple ways you can touch a patient. For example, if a patient tells you that she has had a loss in the family, send out a sympathy card. Keep a stack of cards and stamps in the office for such opportunities. It takes two minutes to write the card and put it in the mail. The gesture is unexpected from a dental office, but it makes the patient feel so much closer to, and valued by, the practice.

Give a Call

Some patients require extensive periodontal care that leaves their gums sensitive and sore for the next few days. Always make a note to call and follow up to see how they're doing. Again, it takes a few minutes, but the impact is tremendous. This opens the line of communication even after the appointment and shows that you're still thinking about them, and that you care.

These are all very low-cost or no-cost things that have a huge impact on people. In this day and age, everything is electronic. It's a nice touch to receive a handwritten letter with a postage stamp. Who doesn't like getting mail? (Other than junk mail, of course!)

Stay Social

Now you can also use social media to connect with patients. You can take pictures of them with you while they're at your office (with their permission, of course), and then you can text it to the patient so they have it too. Just taking a picture with a patient makes them feel special.

Always ask to post the picture to Facebook. Chances are, if you send them the picture, they'll also post it to Facebook, and your practice will reach that many new people. The patients who have a great experience always seem to be willing to post on their Facebook page. This is yet another simple strategy to make the patient feel special and increase the success of the practice. Pinging your patients and having them think of your practice will keep you relevant. It is a style of branding your office. You never know who they will meet that needs a dentist. Finding a great dental office is not easy, and patients know that. They want to say "MY dental office." They want to know they have a dental home.

Don't Reward Patients for Bad Habits

Ailments such as gum disease can progress further if the patient doesn't take responsibility for their oral health. Part of your job is to correct disease, and that means not rewarding patients for their bad behavior.

The smart way around this is to educate the patient on what it takes to reverse whatever negative things are going on inside their mouth. Some hygienists may be tempted or forced to go overtime to finish a cleaning on a patient who hasn't been properly caring for her teeth. It is better to schedule another appointment and explain to the patient what is going on in her mouth than to throw off the rest of the patient schedule to work around her.

This also empowers the patient. We've talked a lot about empowering the team, but we must also empower the patient. It's great that a patient comes in every three or four months to see you, but what is more important is what she does every day at home to care for her teeth. Make sure each patient understands that even if she comes in for regular appointments, if she doesn't take care of her mouth at home, she will not get the full benefit of what you are providing for her.

This information empowers the patient because she realizes that she plays a huge hand in what happens in the office. It helps her to understand that you are partners in her oral health. But the patient must take responsibility for her daily habits.

Most parents just say to their kids, "Go brush your teeth," and leave their child to it. In fact, there is a very specific way in which people are supposed to brush their teeth. The hygienist has to demonstrate and show the patient, because if the patient isn't shown, she doesn't know.

It's like gaining a coworker. If you have a new team member, the team has to teach her and train her how to do something; otherwise, you can't hold her responsible for something that goes wrong.

The hygienist has to give the patient the tools and the power to be able to implement good oral hygiene on a daily basis. Thus, the hygienist has to come up with a plan for that patient—one with which the patient will actually comply. The hygienist has to be realistic and talk to the patient to gain this understanding. Maybe you need to think outside the box in order to come up with a solution. Bottom line, the patient is in your charge. Even after you come up with a plan, you have to follow up with her at her next visit and reassess.

It's important to compliment the patient on any improvement, even if the improvement is very small. Patients don't want to come in every time and be told that their mouths are in poor shape and that they need to step it up. Remember what we talked about in the previous chapter: people like to be around leaders. Leaders make other people feel great about themselves when they are around others. Put yourself in the patient's shoes. Would you want to be told you're doing a horrible job every few months? Do you think that would lead to broken appointments, poor treatment acceptance, and an overall poor outlook in your office? The answer is: *absolutely.*

Even the smallest compliment could be the encouragement a patient needs to keep trying harder. This dynamic will help you gain respect from the patient by being empathetic and sensitive to what that patient individually needs.

Some hygienists are afraid to bring up something they see the patient should be doing because they don't want to offend her. The truth is, there is a way to give advice and gain trust. For instance, you can share with patients how flossing is not just the most important thing that they can do for the health of their mouth, but how flossing is the most important thing that they can do for the general health of their whole body.

Patients are often surprised and want to know more. This gives you the opportunity to talk about the oral-systemic link wherein evidence-based science has found that the bacteria in the mouth are directly related to heart disease. Chances are, you'll enjoy the opportunity to teach and your patients will be happy that now they know something simple they can do for their health.

Establishing trust and prioritizing time with your patients is really not that hard. Now that you have a set of guidelines for establishing good rapport and caring for them in the best way possible, you can begin to transform your relationship at the practice.

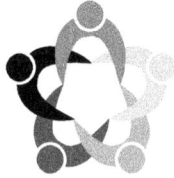

CHAPTER 6

Dear Team Leader:
The Team Depends On You

With Contributions from
Stephanie Curcio, CTF-TC

I n a typical dental office, you walk in and see an over-crowded room with people waiting to get in. If you're lucky, someone greets you at the front desk, or at least nods hello. Or maybe the person at reception is cut off by a glass window or wall, so the room feels more like a holding cell than a waiting area.

By the time your name is called, the dental assistant is frazzled and the hygienist rushes through your cleaning. The dentist takes a quick peek inside your mouth, grumbles something about fillings, and sends you on your way. You walk out of the office feeling like you just got whiplash.

And what do you think? *I need to find a new dentist.*

First impressions have a huge impact on the patient, but the truth is that first impressions are a product of how the practice is functioning as a whole. So much of this first impression begins with the treatment care coordinator. From the first impression to the overall cohesiveness within the team, your role entails a lot of support.

One of the best ways to support the team is to set the tone. That means having the first encounter, when the patient walks into the practice, go as smoothly as possible.

When you walk into a Trust Factor™ office, there's always someone there to greet you, poking her head out, calling you by name. That makes a huge difference for the patient, even if she's new, because she knows that someone is expecting her. You don't get that elsewhere.

The Trust Factor™ practice focuses a lot on eye contact. Get down on the patient's level. Don't disengage in any way, because your focus is to let her know that she has control. To help the patient feel at ease, try your best to say yes to what she has to say.

"Can I have time to think about this?"
"Yes."

"Can I look around?"

"Yes."

"Can I talk to the doctor for an extra minute?"

"Yes."

"Can I ask a couple more questions?"

"Yes. Yes, you can."

Assuming you don't want the patient to walk out or go elsewhere, you say yes, even if the doctor is with another patient. As is the case with many other providers in other offices, once your time with them is done, it's done. You have to come back. The Trust Factor™ office will always make room for a patient because you want her to know that she's special and you care about her—that she's not just another time slot on the schedule.

By establishing that positivity, the patient is primed for the rest of her visit with the team.

Know Your Role

You can support your team by making it clear what each member's role is in the office. In the Trust Factor™ office, there is a dedicated space for everything. In particular, you have a New-Life Room, which is the only room where finances or money for treatment is discussed.

Oftentimes, the dentist is not only the one diagnosing and treating the patient in other offices, but he's the ones going over the money, and that's not the dentist's job. The dentist's job is to treat people. When a doctor is speaking to patients about money, the level of trust is not there and cannot be leveraged. The treatment coordinator (TC) has a higher position on the trust ladder, allowing the TC to be more effective.

The treatment coordinator is the person who's going to get the patient financing. She's the person to whom a patient can direct questions about interest payments. In turn, the coordinator has questions of her own: "Do you know what you need? Do you know what you want? Who do you want to be? What do you want for yourself? What do you need for yourself?"

By asking these questions, people will let you know right away what they need.

Most people are used to assuming the dentist is the one who is in charge, which is not how the Trust Factor™ office operates. You can redirect the patient to the appropriate resource to avoid this confusion. You might see a patient walk over to the doctor's office or ask him a question such as, "How much is this going to cost me?"

Take the initiative to reach the patient and provide her with answers. You can say something along the lines of, "Oh, I'll go over that with you. That's my job. The doctor's job is to worry about your teeth."

The patients are often very surprised to hear that. Often, they're excited because it's different and something they haven't experienced. Patients want the doctor to worry about their health, and they want the treatment coordinator there to worry about anything financial.

I wouldn't want my surgeon, who's overseeing my health care, to have money on his mind when he's performing procedures. All I would be able to think would be, "Oh God, I owe this person $100. Is he mad? Is this going to affect my health care?"

By having two separate people in two separate places, it allows the patient to relax and the dentist to focus on her care, which is precisely what each person needs to do.

Separate the Space

In every office there's an old storeroom filled with junk that's just begging to be utilized.

What can you use it for?

A New-Life Room.

As you might imagine, the New-Life Room doesn't have to be big, but it does have to be welcoming. The benefit of having a larger room is that it can double as a meeting space for the team to discuss things for the day.

When you set up the New-Life Room, put in comfortable touches to make it seem more relaxing for the patient, whether it's a lit candle, or a little lavender in the room. Those small things make people feel instantly relaxed and takes some of the pressure off a potentially stressful conversation.

Another comforting gesture is to keep all tools used for the consultation within clear view of the patient. If you're reading numbers off a computer screen, turn the screen so the patient can see everything you see. The patient will appreciate that openness, and will find it easier to trust the team.

Transform Your Office

The reason people don't follow the trust method is because they go according to what they've seen or what they've been shown. To think outside the box and to do something completely different that is unexpected is what makes you extraordinary. And the Trust Factor™ office does just that. In fact, it strives for that.

What can you do today to make this patient's day different? This person has experienced ten previous consultations. What do you have to offer her that she hasn't experienced?

The answers to these questions come from listening to the patient, asking questions, and switching things up a bit.

Don't be scared to have a little fun. Don't be afraid to laugh. Don't be too timid to ask a person about her family, or her job, or her hobbies, or her interests. When you first bring the patient in for the consultation, money is one of the *last* things to discuss with her, if necessary. Money doesn't come until the end. First and foremost, you have to get to know your patient as a person. Sometimes people just don't seem like they care enough about the person who's in front of them, but the treatment care coordinator should.

Create the Vision of an Empowered Practice

You have to have a clear vision of what you want and then go after it. You cannot expect your patient to sign up with you and have hope and faith that you're going to do a good job and change her life if you can't do something as simple as change your office around a little bit to make the experience better. Positive change leads to success. It leads to optimizing all these results. It leads to cases being accepted.

I want to be able to give other treatment care coordinators the tools, the motivation, and the enthusiasm to get up and say, "OK, I'm going to be different and here's what I'm going to do to get there."

The doctor can help by, that's right, trusting the team. If you're the doctor, allow the team to help you. After all, why have you hired help if you're not letting anyone help you? It's very hard to self-reflect, but as a provider or a dentist, you write down what your needs are, you look at your team, and you say, "I can't do it all. I can't be it all. I'm not perfect. No one is perfect." And the team can fill in.

You have a team who's around you. They're dying to step in to help, get their hands dirty, and interact—not only with the patients, but also with you. If you show them that you trust them, they will do anything and everything to work their hardest for you, and be loyal to you. This will not be just a job for them; it will be a career. These are the people who are going to stay late. These are the people who are going to show up early. These are your team members who are going to go the extra mile for you.

Why would you not want that? Why wouldn't you do everything and anything you could—even though it's hard sometimes—to make that change for your office? When you look at it that way, I don't know a single person, or a single dentist, who wouldn't jump on that in a heartbeat—unless he or she likes self-destructing or simply wants to stay the same.

This isn't just about changing the lives of patients. Because they're not the only ones who are important and deserve it. You deserve it too. Why did you get into health care in the first place? You did it because you wanted to help people.

I've heard a dentist's stress level is right up there with someone who is going through a divorce. But it doesn't have to be like that. Who would sign up for that? No one. If you take control and do those little things we've mentioned throughout this book, it can be so rewarding. Not just for you, but for your team, too.

You want people to leave your practice smiling. Don't just let that be your patients, let that be your team, your coworkers, and yourself.

It makes me so happy so when I see the dental assistant smiling or giggling. It thrills me when I see dental hygienist feel empowered because she educated eleven patients that day. It delights me to see the dentist feel like he's empowered his team, and they worked as hard as they could because they wanted to, not because they had to.

To be a part of a Trust Factor™ team is huge. And it just takes little simple steps. Little details. Opening your eyes and taking a look around to change something that you see isn't quite working for you.

If you can do something that's not only going to increase your happiness, but is also going to increase the dollars in your pocket while making you and others happier, why not do it?

Let us show you what those things are. We've been doing this. We know what needs to be done and we have focused on this for a very long time. Read on to let us teach you what to do and how to try it.

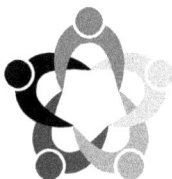

CHAPTER 7

Dear Team Leader:
The Patient Depends On You

With Contributions from
Stephanie Curcio, CTF-TC

Although the treatment coordinator (TC) is the person with the least physical contact with the patients, the TC is probably the most connected from a mental and emotional standpoint. As a result, the TC must have clear perceptions so that the patient understands that the TC is empathetic.

Sometimes, the people who want to hide and disappear are really people who want to shine and be found. So how do you follow your instincts with people?

How do you "read" a person?

And by "read" a person, we don't mean figuring out whether or not he or she has the funds. Instead, other than money, what's holding someone back from the treatment he or she needs? Lack of trust? Fear?

What's the driving force? What's the personal motivator?

In this chapter, you'll learn how to determine just that. I'll share with you how to connect with all different types of people, and how that connection can empower your patient and give her hope.

You see, empowerment begins with hope. Patients come in with so many different scenarios and conditions, but the main reason they come to us is so we can give them hope that they will be OK. As a Trust Factor™ team, it is our role to paint the vision of the future for the patient so that she can see it for herself. If she sees the vision of how her life will change, she will be more likely to say yes to her treatment.

Patients need to be told that we're on the same team. If you're a treatment care coordinator, then you are a people-oriented person. You relate to the patient on a very emotional level, so your goal is to show her that she is not alone.

The first goal is to discover what it is that connects you, specifically, to the patient and from then on, be a guide to let her know that she can make positive changes.

At the same time, you have to be honest. The patient has to know that if she doesn't make the changes, she may truly be hurting herself. It's a fine balance, one that requires candor and tact, but learning how to communicate on an honest, open level with the patient will ultimately win her over.

Here are a few strategies for navigating that balance in your office:

1. A Good Dose of Laughter

In all situations, laughter is the best medicine. Use laughter as a tool to communicate that you're happy the patient is at your office. It also conveys that you enjoy working there and that it's the best place for the patient, as well.

2. Open Your Ears

Sometimes, the best thing to say is nothing at all. Sometimes, you just have to listen.

When you listen to the patient and are asked a question, make your answers concise. In a medical scenario, there may be a lot of scary new words the patient is hearing. The jargon can be overwhelming.

Being short, sweet, and to the point allows you to be thorough and quells many doubts or concerns the patient might otherwise have.

3. *Ask Questions*

A good way to facilitate listening is to ask open-ended questions. By asking simple yes-or-no questions, the kind with short, simple answers, you leave room for silence. Silence is the breeding ground for the patient's doubts and insecurities.

To reinforce the questions, remind the patient why she is at the office. As the treatment coordinator, you want her to hear her personal motivator out loud because if she goes off track, that core need is what will bring her back in.

Restate her personal motivator, ask questions about how she feels regarding her treatment plan, and be a careful listener. It's a make-or-break move when it comes to treatment coordinating.

Talking Numbers

"What's this going to cost me? How is this going to affect me?"

Those are the first questions a patient has after her consultation. That's where you step in. You sit the patient down and go through her entire treatment on a piece of paper. You don't, however, answer anything clinical or health-related because that's not the TC's role.

Take the patient at her word, and ask, "How much are you able to put down, out of pocket, so I know how much financing we should apply for?"

By asking that question, you can see what's available for her and not eliminate your bottom line. You can also make sure that you're very thorough with the patient. Tell her straight up, this is what it costs, this is your treatment, here's what we can do. By doing that, you're not leaving any room for her to doubt you or think that you're keeping anything from her.

Never call the cost for treatment a "bill"; instead, call it an "investment." Her investment will allow her to receive much-needed services and better her overall health.

The next step is to delineate what you are going to do for the patient, what she can expect from insurance, and what the remaining investment will be.

Don't back yourself into a corner. If you're going through your patient's financial options, identify what resources are available from top to bottom. Look at it like a pyramid. The base of the pyramid is her option to pay with cash or a check. The middle of the pyramid is credit. And the top of the pyramid is financing.

Then ask, "Which is the superior financial option? Which one of these are you leaning toward most? What works for you? What can you afford? What can you not afford?"

These are uncomfortable questions for anyone, technically. But if you're not afraid to ask these questions, and you know the right way to ask or word them, then it will increase your case acceptance significantly.

Why? Because you're leaving no room for doubt. People get buyer's remorse when they feel you've left things unsaid. By being thorough and asking the uncomfortable questions, you are eliminating this threat.

One thing to keep in mind is that you can only be as good as your team. If all the steps prior to the patient entering the New-Life Room are not taken, these tools that we are giving you will not work. It is a process that must be followed. Take, for example, the doctor. If your doctor is not able to educate the patient correctly, create a "want," and more importantly, address her concerns, then you have ZERO chance of taking care of finances with her.

Watch the process; when a piece is missing, it is not successful. We can blame the patient and create excuses (which again, are just well-planned lies), but in reality, we, as a Trust Factor™ team, did not exercise our roles as needed.

As you're guiding the patient through her financing options, you want to be aware of what is best for the practice and what is best for the patient, as well as how the two interests can combine.

In any business, cash or check is preferable. However, this is what the patient wants to protect the most. You may find that most patients would like to make monthly payments if possible. They want to retain funding elsewhere as opposed to taking it directly out of their pocket.

In the Trust Factor™ office, you don't want to eliminate other possibilities for the patient in case you can help them. Your objective is to figure out whether or not, if you don't get her the financing (if she, instead, gets a partial loan or captures the full amount), you can fall back on what she said earlier about what is available to her. That way, at the baseline, you have something to work with. A little help is better than none at all.

By setting it up that way and not cutting yourself off, you don't just eliminate the entire treatment plan in itself, but rather, build the foundation to make treatment possible and as worry-free as can be.

Empowering the Patient

When you first bring in a patient, ask yourself:

"What does the patient need from me?"

This isn't solely about medical assistance; this is also about emotional needs. Is the patient soft-spoken? Is she shy? Is she loud? Is she overstimulated?

From there, ask:

"What do I have to offer the patient?"

Maybe she needs tools and resources for financing, or maybe she just needs an open ear. How can you tell unless she specifically says so?

It's in the Way She (or He) Moves

Body language is a powerful communicator. The way you move or hold yourself conveys a lot to the patient.

Similarly, the way the patient physically holds herself is a clue as to what she needs or wants.

There are simple things you can do as far as body language is concerned. Do not disengage with the patient. Show eye contact and keep locked in on the patient. Don't be negative in any way. It's all about internal empowerment.

If the patient is hunched over or stiff, maybe she needs a calming touch on the hand.

If the patient is having trouble making eye contact, then maybe she is nervous and needs you to reassure her.

A lot of patients who come into dentistry have already gone through traumatic experiences. They're in that fight-or-flight mode, and you are in a position to diffuse that anxiety. Physicality can achieve a lot.

Dr. James Dobson, Ph.D., is founder of Focus on the Family, a nonprofit organization that produced his internationally syndicated radio program. On the program, he discusses the twelve steps of intimacy. Although he discusses these steps as they relate to marriages and relationships, they can also be applied to dentistry and the new patient (for the most part). The Trust Factor™ office will use these steps to get to know the patient and earn her trust. Understanding the patient in a process-oriented fashion, as opposed to an all-in approach, will gain that desired trust.

When the Patient Isn't So Receptive

The Trust Factor™ coordinator provides an extraordinary experience for the patient. But that doesn't always mean the patients are extraordinary. Some can be rude, difficult, or downright hostile. Even in these tense situations, you must always comport yourself in the same manner as you would with your closest patient. Kill the anxiety with your kindness.

The patient doesn't expect you to be extraordinary— especially during tense situations. The last thing a rude or a blunt person expects from you, the treatment coordinator, is patience and kindness. But if you are persistent in your patience and kindness, the rudeness tends to diffuse.

It can be hard to sit across from a person who is lashing out at you, but you must maintain the perspective that whatever it is she's going through, it's not you. You can't take it personally.

Quite the opposite—you have to focus even more on what that patient needs.

An overly worried person or someone who's been scarred from her previous dental experience needs to be reassured. She needs kindness, and that needs to come through in the TC's demeanor, regardless of the behavior presented.

Sometimes you have to fight for the patient. By that, we mean, someone who comes across as hopeless or defeated by previous dental experiences needs you to go the extra mile to show that you care about her wellbeing.

Reassure the patient that you're there for her. Tell her not to give up on herself because you're not giving up on her.

The Trust Factor™ office categorizes the patients into groups A, B, C, and D.

The A patient will say yes to whatever you recommend. As the level of trust is so high, no acrobatics are necessary. This patient will be your patient for life.

The B patient has a level of trust, but just wants a little information to validate her decision so that she can be transformed into an A patient. She wants to know what her insurance benefits and finance options are, and then she will say yes.

The C patient is downright hostile. She is rude on the phone, she doesn't open up in the New-Life Room, and she's very challenging. Although the patient is fueled by fear of the unknown, she also may be acting like this because of her previous experience at another dental office.

The truth is that she is just looking for someone she can trust, someone who will listen to her. Following the Trust Factor™ process with her will not only convert her to an A patient, but also turn her into your most vocal advocate. So don't be alarmed by the initial presentation of these patients; in time, they can prove to be your most valuable.

The D patient, on the other hand, is the patient you never had a chance with from the beginning. This is the patient who will never say yes to treatment, never come to her appointments, and will take up 90 percent of your practice time with negativity. Identify this patient and cut the cancer off before it invades your practice.

Sympathy Versus Empathy

It's easy for people to be sympathetic, but there's a very fine line between showing someone sympathy and being empathetic. You want to show the person empathy, not sympathy.

When you tell someone that you feel bad for him or her, you may feel like you're relating, but really, you're showing sympathy and piling on negativity to the experience he or she has gone through.

To be empathetic is to be able to relate to that person and say, "Wow, I understand what you felt in that moment. I've been there. I went through something similar to that myself. I want to be there with you while you go through this." It's more about being a guide than being one who pities. Empathy is proactive; sympathy is destructive.

By listening and knowing the difference between the two, you become a huge asset for the team. In fact, the whole team should understand the difference between sympathy and empathy. Each person touches the patient and has a hand in educating. If everyone knows how to focus on a proactive approach to relating to patients' negative experiences, then you can make a positive difference in their lives.

The Five-Year Technique

If you're still having difficulty conveying the importance of treatment to the patient, use the Five-Year Technique.

Ask the patient, "Where will you be in five months if you didn't come here today?"

"What about five years?"

This helps the patient to visualize herself. If you found an infection, ask her to imagine what it will be like in five months when it's over and she is finished healing. Can she see herself in that light?

When a person sees that picture, it reassures her why she's in the office in the first place. Remember, we are not treating teeth; we are treating people. Your job as a Trust Factor™ office is to paint the vision. Paint the picture. Show her what is possible. The better your painting, the higher the success you will have as an office.

There are a lot of patients who are very jaded by the trauma they've experienced, or the bad experiences that they've had as children, or in their past with other care. Redirect that negativity into positivity.

Remind the patient that her painful experiences allow her to change her life. Don't waste time with regret. That's in the past. She is more valuable than that.

When a person hears that she's valuable, that she doesn't have to live life in pain or with the belief that she deserves poor treatment, she feels incredibly empowered. Ask her power questions, like "What can we do for you to have it all now?"

Being Open

We want to spend a moment to build on our point that honesty and thoroughness are the best policies. Openness and honesty are the two best *tools* for creating the treatment plan with the patient. Being direct, but not condescending or rude, is so appreciated. We are at a place in the world where we have so much information right at the click of a button, through technology, via cell phones, and on TV.

Often, patients will have already Googled and researched everything on dental implants and Invisalign®, and know the cost and what to expect. But what they don't expect, and what you can't research, is the experience. So that's what you're selling them. You're selling them your family. You're giving them the opportunity to better their lives.

Patients come to you with questions. Some patients want a second opinion; some just want to be out of pain, but if you withhold information and you're not thorough, then it looks as if you have something to hide. And you don't.

I remind myself to not be afraid to state, or ask, the patient the obvious.

Even if the information is stated on a piece of paper that they've signed to accept treatment, you want to be certain that she fully understands everything. If there's fine print at the bottom that you have not explained, a person will feel betrayed later on when she reads through it on he own and you're not around to answer questions. Of course, it was never your intent to pull the wool over your patient's eyes, but that's how she will view it.

A lot of treatment coordinators view their job as getting the patients to case acceptance and securing money. This conception is only holding them back. The very questions that they should be asking, they're afraid to ask. The conversation they should be having, they're *not* having.

Treatment care coordinators don't ask the necessary questions due to a fear of rejection. People don't want any negativity directed back towards them in any way. This fear comes from taking things too personally.

Accepting the Case

If the patient needs time to think, I always make a follow-up call to review everything we discussed during the appointment. If she needs a second consultation simply to go over everything again, or to have her partner in on the decision-making process, then happily schedule that.

Many times, however, the patient will accept it right then over the phone because you've shown that you're willing to work with her. You've shown that even after she has left the office, you're still thinking about her.

There are a small percentage of patients out there for which there's nothing you can do or say that will inspire them to accept treatment. These are the people who have quite often been to a dozen other consultations. They've been told what's going on, and it's not a matter of fear; it's not a matter of trust. It's just that they don't get treatment because it's what they've chosen to do.

When we're talking about a care coordinator, we're talking about one who creates an emotional bond with the patient. We're not just trying to sell her services; we're also trying to become a trusted advisor to her. My hope for all the patients who are avoiding treatment, is that they connect with someone who has read this book and can get through to them so they know how important their oral health is to their overall health, and how a dental practice can transform their life.

So let's talk more about transformation in the office. If you're a dentist reading this, and you want to implement these changes and empower the patient, what do you do?

First step: Get your team together.

Gather together your team members, go to the front door, and walk through your office. See it through a new patient's eyes. Then discuss. What do you see when you walk through the door? What attracts you? What distracts you?

Do you have wires hanging around the office? Is it dirty? Do you have refreshments out for the patients to make them feel more comfortable? Is your receptionist greeting the patients? Are you smiling? Are there papers everywhere? Are there materials there to educate the patient on what services you offer? Are your accolades up on the wall?

It's in the Details

You want to walk into a place and know that that person has studied his specialty. You want to know that he has continued his education and that he loves what he does. In the traditional office, you would call this entry room the "waiting room." Instead, call it the "Hospitality Room."

Don't say, "Come to the reception area." Instead, that's the "Greeting Area." Nor should you refer to the patient's time as an appointment. It's a "visit." Those little shifts in vocabulary are huge.

If you haven't picked up on it already, all of these changes that you can make to keep your patients happy provide a good deal of happiness for the team too. It's not difficult to empower your practice because, once you begin, the satisfaction it brings is infectious. Take a moment to look at what the finer details of your office say to your team and your patients. Identify ways that you can increase the happiness factor with a few small touches!

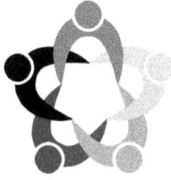

CHAPTER 8

Four Cubits to Succeed

The Trust Factor™ office is slow to hire and quick to fire. We have conducted many interviews with many candidates. At this point, we've seen it all. We once interviewed a candidate who wanted a job in exchange for an exorbitant amount of money. She had been working in an office for nine years and had lots of experience. We asked her how many people were working in her office.

She said, "Well, there's the doctor, the hygienist, and me."

We asked, "You've been working there for nine years?"

Again, she nods.

"Why hasn't the practice grown in nine years to require more members?"

She looked at us, dumbstruck.

This young woman obviously was not happy at the practice where she had spent nine years of her life; otherwise, why would she be looking for a job at our office? The growth (or lack thereof) of her former office was only proof of that discontentment.

The team grows your practice. The way for that to happen is for the team to take ownership. The way for the team to take ownership is for you to stay within your "four cubits."

What does that mean? Stick with your expertise; focus on your job and let your team members shine in theirs.

Staying within your four cubits is the same as what my teammates have said throughout the book: *Doctors, you need to let go and trust.*

If you set up strict guidelines and rules, and micromanage your team, then they are not going to enjoy working with you. It's unlikely that they will grow your practice, and highly likely that they will end up like this young woman— searching for another position. Train your team members so well that they can leave, but treat them so well that they won't *want* to leave.

On the other hand, if you allow your teammates to take ownership of the office, to imagine it their house, then they will treat it like their house—like their baby.

Your dental office is your home, whether you're an assistant, a hygienist, a doctor, or a treatment coordinator. You spend most of your time in within those four walls, and so everyone should feel as if he or she has ownership of that space.

When It's Time to Make a Change

Many people have difficulty identifying when change is necessary. Often, this realization comes too late, after years of flat-line growth and staggering team-member turnover. So how do you know?

When you start to have revolving doors of employees and patients, then it's time to pump the brakes. It's time to accept the idea that maybe the problem isn't everyone around you; maybe the problem is you.

Our practice doesn't run perfectly. We work hard every single day and are constantly encountering obstacles to work though. The difference between our team and most other practices is that we say, "Hey, if we hit a roadblock, let's stop what we're doing and tackle this together."

Like we said at the beginning of the book, I am not the Lone Ranger. We need our team if we want to be successful.

I learned my lesson the hard way. I bought a dental practice in 2007, and I immediately lost 30 percent of the patients within six months.

Why? Because I came in and said "I am Dr. Jon. I'm the boss. I'm gonna do what I need to do, and if you don't like it, you can leave. Whether you're an employee, whether you're a patient, this is the way it's gonna be."

I ran the practice like a dictatorship. I told myself I didn't need that 30 percent. I brushed it off and said, "Whatever. I can't make everybody happy."

Then the year 2007 became 2008, and by 2009 I realized, "Whoa. I'm making money. But I'm not growing, I'm stagnant. Why?"

I wasn't happy with my day-to-day job functions. I was treating people who weren't grateful, and that's not fun to wake up to every single day. Our profession is hard enough as it is. When I left my home to go to my second home, I didn't want to feel like I was walking on eggshells because my team—who I treated more like my "staff" at that point—didn't trust me.

I realized the team was reacting to my energy. In turn, patients reacted to that energy. Finally, I was brave enough to say, "Hey, let me step back for a second. Why is it that this person has such an amazing practice? I'm a better dentist than he is, but when I see him at a trade show, his team is so happy."

It's because he gives his team members validation, and they give their patients validation. The doctor stayed within his four cubits and respected his teammates to perform their jobs and take responsibility.

The doctor ran a Trust Factor™ office.

When I made this connection, there was no turning back. I wasn't about to wait another moment, let alone a year, to transform my practice.

Perhaps you can relate. My guess is that you didn't buy this book because you're happy with where you are. You bought this book because you're at a point where you need to grow.

You need to change something in your life, and it may not have anything to do with money. It may just be that you want to feel more fulfilled. If you're a dental assistant and you bought this book, it may be because you've been to so many offices and you're tired of it.

What do you need to do to be able to enjoy your job?

You can be in denial and say your hang-up is everybody else's problem, or you can look inside and figure out what you can change.

What can you do to make people really want to be around you? That's how we get patients to stay with us. That's how we get employees stay with us. That's how we get dentists stay with us.

Successful people don't say, "What can people do for me?"

Successful people say, "What can be done for others?"

Every day in the Trust Factor™ practice, we ask what we can do for others. We try our best to work with each other, and work with the community to care for each other.

Once I was doing a reconstruction case with surgery and everything ended up taking a little bit longer than I thought. I was working into lunch and I was focused, and my assistant came to me and said, "Dr. Jonathan, put it down."

"Put what down?" I asked, distracted.

"You need to stop," she said. "I'm going to do this for you, and you just go sit down. Because you can't keep going like this."

She could have easily taken her lunch break, but she cared enough to check on me. When she saw I was working hard, perhaps too hard, she tapped my shoulder and stepped in for me. Why? Because she knew that I would do the same for her. The whole team knows. We help each other because we are connected. Although I've learned to stay within my four cubits, it empowers my team to better know my needs and feel confident to step up.

When you have Trust Factor™ team members who feel that connection at the practice, that energy is transmitted to the patient. Even though the patient might be in the chair and can't speak, she can hear and feel everything. Those small exchanges make a huge impression.

Whether you took out four of her wisdom teeth, performed implant surgery, or did a root canal, she's still going to walk out and be impressed. Even though the dental work may have been painful, all she will remember is that the assistant was smiling the whole time.

No one goes into dentistry just to scrape teeth. And if that's how you view your job, you are not going to be happy.

If you went into dentistry to be able to be the gatekeeper of the patient's health and make changes in the patient's life, then this will be the best job in the world.

I've been trash-talked before about my profession. I've been told that I'm not a real doctor. My hygienist has been told she's just a gum gardener, and my assistant, that she's a spit sucker.

Well, the people who say that really have no idea what we do. But the patients know, and they value us. If your doctor is a Trust Factor™ doctor, then you will never work for anyone; rather, you will work with people who empower you to be your best.

It requires the whole team to change the way that you look at things. You have to understand that every person who is in those four walls is there for the patient. It is a job, but it's also a form of philanthropy. It brings joy to other people's lives, and in turn, to one's own. The greatest joy in the world for my team is to be able to give to someone else. That joy has no price on it.

Throughout these pages, you've gained insight into the roles and responsibilities of the key players in my office. You've learned how important it is for each member to feel empowered, and how that empowerment stems from trust in others to do what they do best.

By staying within my own four cubits, I do what I do best—dentistry—and I allow my team to flourish. Ultimately, this is what has made the difference between flat lining in 2009 versus the tremendous growth I now experience each year. It's the Trust Factor™ difference, and the power is real.

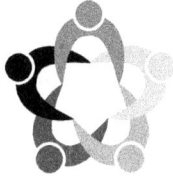

CHAPTER 9

Create the Experience

When we talk about how to get the patient to want to see you, it's really the last step in the whole process. The fact is, if you trust your team, if you empower each member of the practice, then you won't have to worry about how to get your patients to want to see you. That part will just come naturally.

The success of your practice really comes down to the aura—that impalpable energy that can't be seen, but can most definitely be felt as soon as the patient walks into the office.

So how do you establish that aura?

You make the office feel like home.

If you're a team member and you're reading this, then your job is to feel that you're an important part of the practice, like this is your office. You may be the treatment coordinator, hygienist, or assistant, but the practice is equally your home.

Imagine inviting someone into your home. Of course you want to make him or her feel comfortable and welcome, but how do you do that? You set the mood, you fill it with joyful reminders of what you love, you create a zone of happiness.

"Make yourself at home," you say, because you know that this will make your guest feel most comfortable. The last thing you want your guest to feel like is just that—a guest.

The Trust Factor™ practice is a home for all who enter. When you come into the dental office, the first thing that you see is a smiling face, and that's a *real* smiling face—somebody who is really happy, not somebody who tells you to sign in and shuts the window. Not someone who says, "We'll be with you in a couple of minutes . . . " and they make you wait forty-five minutes.

When a patient comes in, she senses that you are inviting her into your home. As a result, she feels welcome and she wants to be there. She wants to spend the rest of her life coming to your office to have you take care of her dental health.

It's a very simple concept, making the dental practice the team's second home, and yet very few people run their practice this way. And guess what—more and more offices are shutting down. More and more offices are not achieving the success they desire.

Dentistry is a wonderful profession. It's not that hard to make a living as a dentist; you just have to have the right people and take pride in what you do. But if you come in every single day, and can't wait to clock out, then why would anyone want to work for you, or *with* you? Why would anyone want to go to you for your services?

Patients come to the Trust Factor™ office after having miserable experiences with other offices. I always ask, "Why did you leave?" The reasons vary, but it's always something along the lines of "They weren't nice," or "They didn't listen to what I wanted," or "They didn't care about my needs."

On the other hand, I encounter many dental professionals who can't wait to leave their current office. The number one reason a team member leaves a dental office is because she wasn't validated. She wasn't told that she was important and she felt limited in her role.

The mistake that many dentists make is thinking that employee satisfaction comes down to money. Truly, it is not about the money. When people feel great about what they do, feel that they're making a difference, feel that they're leaving a legacy—that's what job satisfaction is all about. And that job satisfaction attracts patients.

Connecting to Your Community

Being a dentist means playing an integral role in your community, whether you recognize it or not. You have the ability to touch people's lives when they walk through your door. That's an opportunity to both appreciate and take advantage of.

I recently had a patient come in who hadn't been to the dentist in years. His teeth were broken and I knew it would take a lot of work to make his smile right again. I thought, *This is your opportunity to help him.*

You would think, *What is he doing with his teeth?* You might also want to ask him that question, but you have to stop and consider: What did it take for him to actually walk through those doors?

When he first came in, he felt so vulnerable. He didn't even look us in the eye when we tried to talk to him; that's how embarrassed he was. On top of that, he didn't have good credit, and he had very little resources. He wasn't even sure he could get the help he needed. So we worked extra hard to get him approved for a very minute amount of money.

When I first sat down to talk to him, I asked, "What do you do for a living?"

He said that he was retired and had a limited income. He had a set amount of money to invest in his mouth. It wasn't a lot, but it was enough for us to be able to change his life. He was a C patient with a specific need. Now his mouth is beautiful, which gives him confidence as a retiree. And now he's a patient for life. Guess what—he referred his wife and his daughter, who are now a part of our Trust Factor™ family.

I could have said to him, "Listen, the treatment is this amount, and if you can't come up with this number of dollars, leave." Plenty of other dentists had done so. That's what I probably would have done in 2007 when I first bought a practice and ran it for all the wrong reasons. But when you're able to listen to people and truly make an effort to serve them, at the end of the day, you make the money and you change lives.

That gentleman has gone on to send us new patients, who, in turn, send us more new patients. It's a circle that just keeps growing—a circle in which you're enriching people's lives. And that's the best feeling you can have when you go home at five o'clock.

Don't Nickel and Dime

Most dental offices work based on ADA procedure code. You need a cleaning? The code is this. You need an extraction? The code is this. You need ten extractions? The code times ten. It's like ordering a hamburger and French fries at a fast-food restaurant; you can see each item ticked on the screen, along with the grand total.

The Trust Factor™ office does it differently. The Trust Factor™ practice charges a comprehensive price for the comprehensive treatment patients receive. If the services were itemized, it would cost so much more money for the patient and compromise their trust. This way is much simpler and mutually beneficial.

Patients are informed of this so that they can understand that if something changes during the procedure, they won't be charged more or less for anything. They appreciate the service and especially the discount they are receiving. This builds trust with patients that you are not going to over-charge them like their handyman or any other service they may receive.

Imagine you're performing comprehensive care and you tell the patient that it's going to cost a certain amount. Then you actually do the procedure only to realize that you didn't account, for example, for a bone graft in the final bill. Are you going to stop the surgery, sit the patient up, and ask her to authorize an extra $1,000–$1,500 procedure?

How would you feel if somebody did that to you?

People may add on expenses all the time in undertakings such as building a house, but this is not construction.

You're a health-care provider, and your billing methods should reflect that.

Of course, it would be false to say that there isn't a business transaction involved with dental work. But there's a difference between charging for your services versus nickel-and-diming for your services. This requires a great deal of treatment-planning skills on the part of the doctor. With today's diagnostic methods and CE training, the Trust Factor™ doctor can attain the level of expertise to not make a mistake.

In the Trust Factor™ practice, we live by a book called *The Four Agreements by Don Miguel Ruiz.* The book outlines four values by which you should model your life:

1. **Be impeccable to your word.**

   If you give your patient your word that you're going to provide for her, then never go against it.

2. **Don't make assumptions.**

   Don't assume that someone is going to say something or do something or feel something. If you have a question, then ask. Don't assume, based on the patient's excuses why she can't pay for the dentistry, that she doesn't deserve the most comprehensive care. Diagnose to give the patient the best, not to provide what her insurance or "alleged wallet" has in it. Allow the patient to make her own decision about what she wants. Your job is to *share* the information.

3. **Don't take anything personally.**

    Always maintain patience and understanding, and in those moments when you feel like you might lose your cool, try to see it from the patient's perspective.

4. **Always do your best.**

    Maybe the patient is acting a certain way because she's afraid and she's just putting on a "tough guy" attitude as a front. Don't say, "Well, this lady didn't pay me as much, so I'm not going to do as good at my job." Always do your best. Always treat your team the best because if you don't treat them great, then they are not going to treat you great. When you show a patient that you're going to do all four of these things, then nothing can stop you.

What these four agreements underline is the ability to understand the patient. Understanding what's special for her. Understanding what she goes through. The same goes for your team.

Everybody is wired differently, and not everybody can be treated exactly the same way. Some people just work because they want a job, and no matter what or how you speak to them, they're always going be there. But you want to be around inspiring people because you're inspirational. You have a hand in changing people's lives, and your team allows you to do it. You're never going to be the artist if they don't get you the canvas and paintbrush and paint to make it all happen.

Your canvas is your patient. Your team could sabotage that canvas by making the smallest of errors, such as not answering the phone correctly. When the patient comes in, they could be rude to her. They could prejudge the patient.

There's so much financial loss going on in your practice because your team members are not doing what they're supposed to be doing. And the reason they're not doing what they're supposed to be doing is because *you're* not doing what you're supposed to be doing.

You need to create a vision. Have a vision for what you want for yourself in the next five years, and have those people be in the vision with you. It all goes back to the rowing analogy. If you have ever watched rowers, the way they row, they have a destination: a straight line. They're going directly from point A to point B, no twists or turns or stops along the way. If somebody's standing at the front telling them which way to go, then they will arrive. But if they're not in sync, what happens to the boat? It goes to the left. In just one stroke, they can completely lose track.

You have to align your team and your oars with the same vision. Get your team on board.

When you can impart to your team members that they're special and that you value them, then the rest—getting patients to *want* to come in—is cruise control.

Patient return rate, new-patient rate—that's the easy part. It's all the work that goes on in the background that's the trick—all the work that we've described leading up to this chapter. That's the important part. And now you can capture it for yourself.

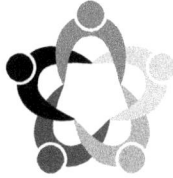

CHAPTER 10

Hey Everyone:
Let's Create a Culture

S uccess in business is not just measured in income or revenue earned, but by how we feel going into work on a daily basis. Having fun and enjoying ourselves, while helping our patients and team members, is the ideal situation for every office, including a dental practice.

When our team members have trust in us, the seemingly endless tasks, responsibilities, and meetings feel more meaningful, which is extremely important when it comes to fostering a supportive and productive office culture.

Essentially, the office culture affects every aspect of your business, and can be the difference between high–functioning and low–functioning practices, which is why it's so important to invest in cultivating a happy and productive culture.

A team culture of trust, fun, and quality work transfers to your clients. One example of strong team culture that is infectious and attracts people regardless of cost can be seen at SoulCycle, the indoor cycling gym. At SoulCycle, the employees are working hard, building relationships with each other and clients, and genuinely enjoying their work. Consequently, clients have a blast, push themselves, and sweat all over the place while being excited and eager to come back for their next workout.

As dentists, one of the most important things that we need to do to ensure success is to create a culture for our selves, our team members, and our patients. It's important to note that you cannot just create this culture for one of the three, it has to be for all aspects of your office: yourself, your team, and your patients.

The Vision

To begin with, you have to create a vision: really visualize what you want to do every day in your practice, then turn that into a statement that you can communicate to your team members and patients. Start by deciding what type of dentistry you want to practice. Do you want to do dentistry that involves working as many hours as possible? Do you want to practice low-end dentistry? High-end dentistry? Insurance dentistry?

Once you decide on the type of dentistry you are going to build your practice around, you can create your vision, and then craft your office culture to support that vision. For example, if your practice focuses on full–mouth reconstruction—the type of dentistry that often changes lives—then you need to be able to change your teammates' lives too. If your team doesn't come in and say, "I'm not here to just punch in and punch out—I'm here to really make a difference in people's lives," then how are they going to be able to impart that passion to your patients?

Once you create a culture for your team that says, "You're here to change lives. You're here to help people," they're going to be happy to be there and they will make sure that your patients know it.

You can tell whether or not your team is happy to be there based on their responses when you ask them to complete a task. If they respond with, "Alright, I'll get to it," then you know that they view the task as an obligation. If the response is more along the lines of, "Sure thing, happy to help," then you know that they feel like they are a part of a team and that they're doing work that makes a difference.

To create this culture, we have to start with ourselves. We have to create a culture that makes us happy to go into the office every day. Then we can extend this culture to our team and to our patients.

Forget the Fear

Many dentists are literally petrified of their patients leaving their office. This fear is paralyzing because it makes dentists avoid talking to their patients about anything uncomfortable. For example, dentists should talk to patients who treat their team members poorly. They should also be comfortable discussing the cost of their services, and refusing a procedure that the patient requests if it isn't to their long–term benefit.

This fear of losing patients creates a culture that acts like the patient is doing you a favor by coming to your office. This should never be the case; you are not indebted to your patients. You are the practitioner. You are the one that spent thousands of hours to get where you are, and you continue to improve your practice and stay up-to-date on dentistry advancements. You are constantly thinking about your practice, your team, and your patients.

Your patients don't know all of this. They assume that you're coming in and trying to get to your next client, and that's it. First, you have to understand that it's okay to want to help people *and* make money. The desire for financial benefits doesn't change the fact that your main focus is still to help people.

By being confident in your skills, experience, and desires, your patients will realize that they're not doing you a favor by being in your practice, and that it's actually a privilege for them to be treated by a caring professional. When they understand that you're really there for them, they're never going to leave your practice because their insurance changed or because you informed them of their treatment options. They're going to do what they can to make sure they continue coming to you. You won't have to work six or seven days a week because your patients will adjust their schedules for you. This all starts with the culture you create, and it's up to you if you want to create a culture where your patients decide when you arrive.

When you have a strong patient base that trusts you, they will change their schedules to match your office hours and they won't break appointments. They will understand that the culture of the office is "I can't wait to be there," as opposed to "My insurance changed. I'm out of here." They will appreciate the time and effort you put in, and feel the value of your work.

Creating this culture will allow patients to understand that they are being treated by a team of professionals that goes through extensive training and continued development. All of this will be apparent by the way the phone is answered, how people are greeted when they come in, that patients are given a hot towel before they leave, and that everyone is happy to do these tasks.

Many dentists allow their patients to control too many components of their practice. It's just a matter of reminding yourself that thanking your patients for coming in is a different mindset than that of thanking them for not leaving. This small adjustment will create a better environment and culture for everyone involved, while allowing you to have fun and make the right decisions, not decisions out of fear.

Making decisions out of fear is relatively common amongst dentists because, in general, dentists are afraid of rejection. There is a big difference between DMDs and MDs because medical doctors have more patients than they have time for, so if a patient leaves their practice, it's actually a win for them. Losing a few patients will not have a great impact on the medical doctor's income.

The number of patients that a single dental practice has is not comparable to that of a medical practice, so losing one or several patients will make a big difference. Dentists perform procedures, so not as many people are in need of seeing a dentist as regularly as the majority of people who visit medical doctors. This is the main reason that dentists are afraid to lose clients, and so they start working on weekends and late into the evening to please patients.

Patch Dentistry

Sometimes a patient will come in and say, "Well, can you just patch it? Just patch the dentistry." From the word "patch," you know that it is not the right thing to do. To truly help your patient financially, and for long-term health benefits, you have to correctly fix the problem.

When you have a tire that's punctured, it's obviously better to replace it than to patch it. You usually can patch it, but you know that the tire will be weakened and the fix won't last very long. It's the same in dentistry.

So many patch patients come to my practice, looking for a quick fix to a long-term ailment. They've gone from dentist to dentist to dentist, and never treated the root of the problem.

We look at the x-ray together, and I say to the patient, "Okay, you spent ten, fifteen, twenty, to probably over thirty thousand dollars on your mouth in the past seven or eight years." People don't usually realize the long–term costs associated with patch–work because the issues arise at different times in their lives.

Once we look at it together, they start to think about the implications of that type of dentistry, and are shocked that they need to spend another thirty thousand dollars to fix it. If they had had the work done correctly the first time, it wouldn't have cost them this much and they wouldn't have been in so much pain.

When patients tell you, "Just patch it," you need to educate them and stick to the vision you created for your practice. If your vision is providing quality care, you can say to your patient, "Actually this is not the way that I do dentistry. The way that I do dentistry is different because I care about you, and I don't want you to have issues in the future, so let's do it the right way the first time." This approach will improve the care you provide while strengthening your office culture.

When I bought my practice many years ago, I bought a patch practice. I had patients come in with an amalgam, composite, gold, and gold inlay all in the same tooth, and I patched all over the place. After a while, I decided that I'm not going to have the type of practice that does patch dentistry. There are a lot of patch dentists, but I wanted to differentiate myself as a professional who took pride in his work, did his best for his patients, and practiced lasting dentistry. I was a brand new dentist when I adopted this approach, and I lost 30 percent of my clients within the first three months.

I didn't panic.

Why? Because of the 80/20 rule. This is an idea that I learned from Richard Cost's book, *The 80/20 Principle: The Secret to Achieving More with Less*, which taught me understanding value over quantity when it comes to clients.

In dentistry, we need to embrace that 20 percent of patients are those who keep breaking appointments, only want what is covered through insurance, usually call you on Friday nights for emergencies, and only come in when something hurts—not for preventive care. This 20 percent will make you think that you're making money, but you're actually losing money and your office culture is suffering.

You want to enjoy practicing dentistry, and working Friday nights and weekends won't allow for a healthy work–life balance. We're happy to do it occasionally, but if it's the same 20 percent of patients each time, the patients who didn't listen to our recommendation to begin with, then you have to decide if catering to them in that manner is aligned with your vision.

Instead, focus on the 80 percent of patients who walk into your practice who genuinely want good, comprehensive care. They look to you, the professional, to help them make the best decisions for their oral health. They respect your time, and they respect your opinion.

If you get into the mindset that you only need 80 percent of your patients, then you'll actually be running at 120 percent because the other 20 percent costs you more in the long run.

Another way of distinguishing between the patients to keep, and the patients to let go is to ask yourself: Who are my Ringo Starrs' ? Who are my Waffle Houses?

Your Ringo Starrs are the rock star patients that every dentist dreams of. They're punctual, polite, and are happy to be at your practice. They are the 80 percent.

The Waffle Houses, on the other hand, are a different story. While Waffle House may sound appealing, after you gobble down a greasy, sugary breakfast, you'll regret your decision. Your Waffle House patients make up the 20 percent you'd be better off without. Business—any business—sounds good at the start, but if you choose to work with the Waffle House patients, you will suffer the consequences.

We can't be afraid to let go of that 20 percent of patients who are late, cancel at the last minute, complain about cost, threaten to leave, and so on. The people that are not happy to do the work you recommend, cost you money because their attitude affects other patients and your team. Having a positive mindset means not compromising on your work out of fear, and that's the only way to surround yourself with positive team members and clients. Let go of the Waffle Houses and usher in the Ringo Starrs!

Culture is infectious—the proof is in the pudding, as with SoulCycle. People on bicycles may be pedaling and staring at thirty people in front of them who are sweating, but they're smiling and they're happy to do it. When you walk out of SoulCycle, or any of those great places that make you feel amazing, you recommend it to everyone and are eager to return.

We have to make our dental practice the same: everyone has to be happy to be there. We all have difficult days at times, but we need to put that aside when we go to the office because the culture in your practice defines who you are, how you do business, and the type of patients you have.

People always ask me, "How do you have all these patients? How do you get these cases?" I respond the same way each time: People don't mind the cost because of the value, and they trust me because of the culture of my practice.

Patients know they need the care, so they just want to make sure that you're there for them. Once your patients understand that you aren't just there for yourself, the money will come.

There will be that 20 percent that is always looking for the patch regardless of what and how you explain it to them, but if you make the decision that that's not the type of dentistry you practice, then it doesn't matter if you lose the "Waffle Houses" of the world. You will be gaining more "Ringo Starrs" in the long run.

Culture of Trust

Creating the dental practice that you want is simple. You just have to start from the beginning. People start by going to lectures, workshops, and lessons. They'll take a course on how to place the most beautiful veneers, but that's a waste of time and money until the culture in their practice is healthy. If the culture in their practice is broken, their patients won't trust them, and they will never get to use those skills. You can spend the money on figuring out the latest techniques but your patients will never ask you to perform them if there is a lack of trust.

The key is to focus on having fun. Doing what you love with people that love what they do creates an environment of trust that ensures the success of your business. Once you're confident and not afraid of losing money, you're able to practice the dentistry that you want.

One tool that I use in my practice is a simple piece of paper. When patients agree to a treatment plan, they write their name and date on the sheet, then the fee that is associated with the treatment. The next line states whether the patient is paying with cash or check, and lastly it states, "I'm excited to have a healthy smile." We ask patients to check the box beside that statement in front of us because if they're not excited to have this treatment, then we've failed. They will go home, call to cancel, and ask for a refund. If they're not excited to get this done, and we didn't create that feeling of trust and excitement, then we don't have that culture that makes people look forward to coming back.

Innovative Dentistry and Culture

Dentists are not the coolest people on earth. We're nerds. We love to play with tiny little gadgets and models all day long. We agonize about millimeters and microns, and our office space is a tiny two-by-two-foot square, and we get excited when something changes to a different color or has a better fluorescence.

At the same time, we're also artists, so we have the medical and the creative ingrained in us. We have 3D printers, scanners that take impressions without any goo in your mouth, and in–house milling that can make our crowns the same day. We're using technology creatively in order to take what we do to the next level, and patients love it.

When I teach students in the universities, I'm noticing that the demographic of dentists is changing tremendously. There used to be a stereotype of dentists being sad or having low self-esteem, but it might be because the older dentists created a different culture in their practice, or just used amalgam throughout their careers. What we're doing these days is very different. It's fun and we know that what we do is making a difference for people. It's not that traditional dentistry doesn't make a difference in people's lives, but we are evolving to use more innovative tools and techniques.

It all comes down to your perception of who you are, what you do, and how you help people. The vast majority of us become doctors because we want to help people. If you've become a doctor or dentist to make money, then you're in the wrong profession.

In dentistry, we make a great living, but what we really do is help people. When you help people get from unhealthy to healthy and see them smile, that is worth everything. It doesn't matter if it was that single amalgam they were so self-conscious about whenever they smiled, or if it's their smile reconstruction, or that you gave them brand new teeth to be able to eat again, you're making a difference. You cannot affect this kind of change until you create a culture in your office that makes people want to be there.

You can be flexible, but you have to understand what your vision is for your practice. That way, your patients don't control the hours you work or the type of dentistry you do. No one's going to come into your home and tell you, "Hey, those dishes are ugly. Get another set of dishes because that's what I like." So, why would you allow that in your practice?

Onward and Up: How to Keep Moving Forward

We've targeted the issue and proposed the solution. Now, once you create and implement the vision and culture of what you want, how do you avoid backsliding?

If someone comes in and wants his tooth patched, it seems like you're basically sending money out the door if you refuse. When patients like that come in, you just need to be primed and ready to educate them.

Dentists need to remember that patients don't really know anything about dentistry. Medical doctors don't know anything about dentistry. The general public knows nothing about dentistry. People come to your office because you're the expert, and when they ask for a patch, it doesn't really mean they want a patch. They just don't understand that a patch means that there's going to be a crack left in the tooth and then there's the possibility that they'll have to remove the whole tooth. They don't know that patch–work can do more harm than good, so it's your job to educate them on the problem, the possible consequences, and the solution.

Here's an example of your conversation with a patient, "Let's talk about the problem. The problem is that you have a hole." Begin by validating what patients say is the reason that they came in. Don't dismiss them as being ignorant.

Tell them that you're going to take pictures of their teeth, then follow up with, "I understand that you say you want to patch it, so let's talk about that. Now here's a picture of the tooth, right? You have this hole in your mouth, and here you see this fracture in this tooth? Do you see that?"

If the patient doesn't see it, you can say, "All right, let's take a look at another picture. Do you see it now?"

"Oh no! Is that my mouth?" They are usually shocked when they see what you're seeing.

"Yes." Now you have a captive audience. The idea of patch–work is now slowly going out of the patient's mind. "So, do you know what that crack is?" Now you need to find a way to explain this to the patient without being overly technical. "You know when you get a little crack in your windshield? Have you ever done that on the highway?"

"Yes."

"So, what happened to that crack? Did you fix it right away?"

The patient will say, "Well, I didn't have the chance to fix it. I went to the auto body shop, got a little liquid, and sort of patched that part of the windshield."

"What happened after that?" You ask.

"I kept driving. It got pretty cold, and then the whole windshield exploded, and it was not good. I didn't have my car for a week." This is your opportunity to explain why the patient shouldn't settle for a patch at the moment.

"So that's the same thing that can happen to your tooth, and if you don't have it taken care of, it may happen on a night when you're out on vacation. It may happen when you're out at dinner, and that's the last thing you would want."

You're now explaining the consequences to your patient. So then they'll say, "Well, what's the right thing to do, Doc?" They now understand that you're the expert and they respect your opinion.

Keep in mind that it's important not to dismiss them. Explain to them that you're there to make sure that they don't have any problems. When this is part of your culture, patients will feel taken care of by you, your assistants, the treatment coordinator, and everyone they encounter at your practice.

You create an atmosphere in your practice where the norm is, "This is the place I want to be. I only want to fix it once. I don't want to come to the dentist all the time." You will be surprised at how many people want to have it fixed the right way.

This is similar to Starbucks. Howard Schultz, the CEO of Starbucks, was asked how he gets baristas to smile so much, and he said, "We only hire people who smile." This is the brilliance behind the culture and success of Starbucks: it's not about teaching people to smile, it's about hiring people who smile naturally. Keep this in mind as you hire your team members and as you take on clients.

In order to maintain our vision and culture, we also need to be able to let clients go. We have a culture and we stand by it. In my practice, if we have someone who is the slightest bit mean, I know that they're going to take it out on my team members, and I can't have that. I have to protect my team members from abuse. Zero tolerance for mean people, whether they're on the team or one of our clients. This is very important to protecting your office culture.

If a patient comes in and they're angry, instead of setting fuel to the fire, we diffuse the situation. I say to him, "What's the problem?" If they're upset because their tooth broke, I say, "It's okay. You're in the right place. We're going to help you. You're in good hands today." All of a sudden they just breathe and calm down. People want to know that they're taken care of. All you can do is either diffuse the situation or really add fire to it, so you choose based on what is aligned with your vision.

In my practice, we create a strong culture and then protect it by educating people on why we're the place that they need to be. If they don't move forward right away, it's because they have to work it out in their heads, and that's okay. In the meantime, I'm serving the Ringo Starrs who understand and appreciate what my team and I do, and we're having a blast doing it.

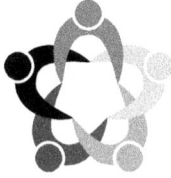

CHAPTER 11

How Can We Brighten
Your Smile Today?

Now that you've read why our process works, it's time to decide how your process will begin.

It starts with a question: What is your vision?

That question expands to: What do you want to grow?

Sometimes those questions are difficult, if not impossible, to answer when you're on the inside looking . . . well, "in."

Perspective is powerful, and that's just what we have to offer. We work with practices to make them excellent using the Trust Factor™ method. Our work is successful not because we create the vision for you; our work is successful because we bring the experience and expertise to work with you to discover just what your vision is. More importantly, we help you put a plan together to make that vision become a reality.

Most dentists don't know where they are going. They don't know what their legacy is going to be. Where do you want to be in five years? Together, let's figure out a way for you to get there.

That's just the beginning—the spark of an idea. That idea becomes a plan, and that plan is backed by experienced professionals who will work with your team. Each one of your team members will be trained by people who have actually practiced dentistry and have lived the trust-empowered experience.

You're going to be trained by people who go through the exact same things that you go through every single day.

The dentist is going to sit with a dentist so they can go through the same challenges together.

The dental assistant is not going to be trained by somebody who's not a real dental assistant. She's going to be trained by actual, working, practicing assistants, so that they can share the same vision. So that she can hear, "You know what? You're not just a dental assistant. You are so much more, too."

Similarly, the hygienist will be trained by a dental hygienist. And the treatment coordinator will be trained by a treatment coordinator.

Why is this process so important? Because the doctor can't be it all. Your team is going to be specialized. The core of what you do will stay the same; you'll still be practicing dentistry and changing people's lives. You'll just do it in a smarter, more successful way—the Trust Factor™ way—that will pave the path for your legacy and enable you to achieve your vision.

By the end of it all, your practice will have that essential quality, that Trust Factor™ "aura" that draws and keeps patients, not to mention, provides the team with an incredibly satisfying and empowering work experience. We'll show you how to get there.

Just as not every patient is right for our dental services, not every practice will be equipped to take on this process. We are looking for those who are motivated, those who want to grow, those who truly want to be happy with what they are doing. We don't accept anything less, and neither should you.

Most importantly, we're looking for people who want to be trained by people who go through exactly what they go through every single day. If you're our match, then you are going to have a tremendous support center. Your practice will transform both clinically and from a management standpoint—two things that very few firms can offer.

Do you want to learn how to do implant surgery? We're going to be your support. You want to learn how to do veneers? We're going to be your support. You have a case that's coming up? You're going to call us.

How are you going to close the case, how do you approach this, how do you do all that stuff? We're going to be that support system based on the vision we create. But it takes a special practice to get started.

This is our legacy; this is how we want to be remembered. We're able to change not only our patients' lives, but we're also able to change our colleagues' lives. For us, it's a win-win situation. Money is not the goal. The goal is to be able to share with everybody and get them to be the best that they can be.

We're not going to tell you who to fire or how you have to take the weight of the world upon your shoulders. Rather, we're going to teach you how to surround yourself with great people. When your team sees that you're investing in a company that believes that they're amazing, that vision is going to come together all the more quickly.

Dentists become dentists because they want to help people. Innately, deep down, they're really good people. I truly believe that assistants and hygienists and people that go into dentistry, it's because they want to help people too. And so the worst thing that can happen to a dentist is when he puts his heart and soul into the process and the patient says, "No." Or the patient says, "I want a second opinion."

It's akin to hearing, "I don't trust you."

When you have the ability to have people trust you because you truly believe in what you're doing, you'll hear a lot fewer of those doubts.

The best kind of dental practice is the one that has the mom-and-pop feel, but you can't run it like a mom-and-pop business anymore. You now have to have business standards, you have to have benchmarks, you have to have people who are willing to make it happen. If you don't have all that in place, then you're going to be gobbled up by corporate dentistry.

Building trust with your patients and your team will allow you to keep going, regardless of the economic climate.

We are so confident in our process that we trust that within one year, you will see results. That is, if you heed our advice and truly want to grow, then you will experience tremendous success.

No matter how long you've been practicing, you'll be excited to come to work every single day, because you're going to be working with people who want to be their best, right alongside you. Dental assistants and hygienists and doctors are all going to want to come to work, because it's a part of their lives. Your office will be a haven, like a protective shield for all of the nonsense that's going on in the regular world.

At the same time, you're going to help change peoples' lives and make more money while working less and doing more of what you want to do. Quite frankly, you may even end up practicing longer because you're having so much fun.

When you change the way you look at things, and change the way you do things, then work turns into fun.

This is why we created the Smile Syllabus Training Institute. The mission of the Institute is to change the face of dentistry. It will host the greatest and most trusted leaders in the industry. We will focus on not only clinical care, but also dentistry from a management perspective. When you attend one of our seminars, you will leave feeling rejuvenated and excited about what lies ahead. So join us on a new journey to discover what dentistry has to offer.

From the second you learn how to treat people, your practice will change. So begin the Trust Factor™ transformation now—and get in touch!

Smile Syllabus Training Institute
1111 Goffle Road
Hawthorne NJ 07506
973-423-4460

www.thetrustfactor.org
www.smilesyllabus.com

www.ingramcontent.com/pod-product-compliance
Lightning Source LLC
Chambersburg PA
CBHW062034200326
41519CB00017B/5030